Communication
for Nurses
Talking With Patients

LISA KENNEDY SHELDON, RN, MS, ARNP, OCN
ST. JOSEPH'S HOSPITAL
NASHUA, NEW HAMPSHIRE

JONES AND BARTLETT PUBLISHERS
Sudbury, Massachusetts
BOSTON   TORONTO   LONDON   SINGAPORE

World Headquarters
Jones and Bartlett Publishers
40 Tall Pine Drive
Sudbury, MA 01776
978-443-5000
info@jbpub.com
www.jbpub.com

Jones and Bartlett Publishers Canada
2406 Nikanna Road
Mississauga, ON L5C 2W6
CANADA

Jones and Bartlett Publishers International
Barb House, Barb Mews
London W6 7PA
UK

Copyright © 2005 by Jones and Bartlett Publishers, Inc.
Originally published by SLACK, Incorporated, © 2004.

ISBN 0-7637-3596-5

Production Credits
Acquisition Editor: Kevin Sullivan
Production Manager: Amy Rose
Production Assistant: Kate Hennessy
Marketing Associate: Emily Ekle
Manufacturing and Inventory Coordinator: Amy Bacus
Printing and Binding: Malloy Inc.

Printed in the United States of America
08 07 06 05   10 9 8 7 6 5 4 3 2 1

DEDICATION

To my parents.

CONTENTS

ACKNOWLEDGMENTS

No book is a solo effort, and particularly not one about communication. While many of my friends, family members, and colleagues have listened to my ideas about a communication text for nursing students, I can only list some of them here. First of all, a thank you to all the people who have allowed me to participate in their care over the years. Your stories have inspired me to think, feel, and understand in ways that have profoundly changed my life. My ability to communicate has changed and is evolving because of each of you. It is an honor to be part of your care.

To my colleagues at work, particularly Paula Drake and Susan Hardy, I appreciate your patience and wisdom, and your wonderful—often humorous—contributions to this book. Thank you to the staff at the Elliot Hospital, Concord Hospital, and St. Joseph's Hospital for being part of the pictures in this book. To Dr. Mary Kazanowski at St. Anselm College, thank you for reviewing this text and providing valuable insight. I am greatly indebted to Judy Sheldon for editing and improving the original manuscript. To the staff at SLACK—John Bond, Amy McShane, Lauren Biddle Plummer, Jim Pennewill, and Robert Smentek—I appreciate all your efforts on behalf of this book. It would not happen without you.

Finally, I want to acknowledge my family—Ray and Louise Kennedy, Margaret Sheldon, Meredith, Laurie, Everett, Zane, Jay, Jamie, Judy, Grace, Paul, and Patty for listening, expressing, laughing, crying, and growing with me throughout our shared lives. To my children, Brad, Greg, Andrea, and Luke, thank you for all the joy you bring to my life. And, finally, to my husband, Tom, I want to express my love and gratitude for your ongoing support and encouragement.

ABOUT THE AUTHOR

Lisa Kennedy Sheldon, RN, MS, ARNP, OCN is an oncology nurse practitioner at St. Joseph's Hospital in Nashua, New Hampshire. She graduated from St. Anselm College with a bachelor of science degree in nursing. After working in a variety of clinical settings, Ms. Sheldon attended Boston College where she obtained a Master of Science degree in nursing as an oncology clinical specialist. Later, she returned to Boston College to obtain postgraduate certification as an adult nurse practitioner. After teaching as a clinical professor at St. Anselm College, Ms. Sheldon returned to the clinical setting in an oncology practice. She has ongoing interests in communication techniques in nursing, particularly to improve patient outcomes and satisfaction. Living in New Hampshire, Ms. Sheldon enjoys spending time with her husband and four children.

INTRODUCTION

CASE STUDY

A 42-year-old man comes to the oncology center to begin chemotherapy for metastatic renal cell carcinoma. The chart says his first name is Edmund and the staff begins calling him Ed. He is a quiet man and often does not share much with the nurses during his weekly chemotherapy. One day, 3 months into his treatment, the nurse is looking at his chart to assess his status prior to beginning chemotherapy. She says, "Ed, I was just looking at your chart and thinking Edmund must be a family name. What do you like to be called?" The patient answered, "Mike. I never liked my first name."

How embarrassing! The staff assumed that he must be called Ed. It would have taken only a moment during the first visit to find out what he wanted to be called.

Small mistakes take place every day when communicating with patients. Some are as simple as calling the patient the wrong name, and others are more complicated, like not understanding a patient's pain because of cultural differences in the expression of pain. We do not intentionally misunderstand our patients, nor do we want to hurt them. It takes a few minutes a day to not only improve how well we talk with our patients, but also how well we listen to what they are telling us. We will better understand our patients' experience, set more realistic goals, and plan more appropriate interventions.

Becoming better communicators means changing our ability to relate to people. I want to relate your communication skills to a geographical situation. In Japan there is a beautiful mountain, Mount Fuji. Not only is it picturesque, it is also where three of the earth's tectonic plates meet and collide, causing earthquakes. Many buildings have been "seismically retrofitted" to be not only functional, but to also withstand the earth's forces. Some have deeper pilings into bedrock, and others have sliding plates to allow the building to move during seismic activity. Your communication skills may be functional, even admirable, but they need to be able to withstand the forces that will challenge them every day. Perhaps a deeper understanding of your values or more flexibility in discussing sensitive issues will enhance your ability to listen and respond to your patients. If this book can "retrofit" your communication skills with a good foundation and techniques that withstand the stressful health care environment, then you will be not only a good communicator but a solid and professional human being. You will know your professional and moral obligations, your own values and personality, and the resources available to provide information and a foundation.

Many of the techniques discussed in this book are meant to enhance professional and personal development. This book takes a closer look at patients and nurses as people and at the ethical, legal, and professional guidelines for communication and nursing interventions. A detailed chapter reviews the therapeutic nurse-patient relationship from the beginning through the actual provision of nursing care and, finally, to the closure of the relationship. Interviewing skills are reviewed as a science and an art with case studies.

Next, the book examines communication with specific patient populations and situations. How do you deal with a patient in a crisis situation? How do you communicate with an intubated patient? What is the best way to give constructive criticism to a colleague? These are a few of the topics that provide practical approaches to difficult communication situations. They are intended to serve as guidelines during times when you are "at a loss for words." With time and experience you will grow into the nurse and communicator you want to be. A nurse can be respectful, caring, funny, sensitive, insightful, precise, concise, empathetic, spiritual, inquisitive, logical, gentle, and peaceful. Each nurse is a unique mixture of many qualities. The development of your communication style is up to you.

Setting the Stage for Effective Communication

Section

1

Chapter *1*

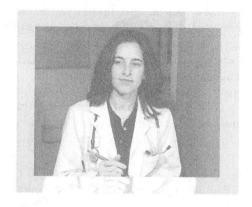

THE FIRST ENCOUNTER

CASE STUDY

"Good Morning, Mrs. T. My name is Jay Kennedy, and I will be your nurse today. Is it all right to call you Mrs. T.?"

Mrs. T. is a 76-year-old woman with metastatic lung cancer being cared for by the nurse, Jay. It is her second day in the hospital. She is quiet, giving one-word answers to Jay's questions. She thinks that Jay is too aggressive, making her wash up and scheduling tests for later in the day. Jay is beginning to wonder about why Mrs. T. is reluctant to share more information. When he comes in to bring her morning medications, he says, "Mrs. T., I have your medications." She responds, "What am I supposed to do, take those now just because you say so?"

INTRODUCTION

This situation is so simple and yet so complicated. The tone of the first words sets the framework for the interactions and care that will follow. Each time a nurse meets a new patient, a relationship begins for both the patient and the nurse. However, this is a different type of relationship, because it involves the nurse as a professional health care provider and the patient looking for assistance during a change in health status. Gone are many of the social boundaries that define everyday relationships. Patients may be required to reveal intimate parts of their lives and bodies within a short period of time, or even submit to painful procedures. In order for the patient to feel respected, comfortable, and safe, the nurse must create an atmosphere that puts the patient at ease, allowing revelation, understanding, mutual planning, and actual interventions to take place.

While setting up this relationship in the short time that nurses are allowed today may sound like an impossible task, it is a clinical skill that can be learned. Each nursing student can learn the basic ability of communicating with patients. These skills build on previous experiences and begin a lifetime of learning for the nurse as both a person and a communicator in a professional role.

Communication is a universal word with many meanings. Many definitions describe it as a transfer of information between a source and a receiver. In nursing, communication is a sharing of health-related information between a patient and a nurse, with both participants as sources and receivers. The information may be verbal or nonverbal, written or spoken, personal or impersonal, issue-specific, or even relationship-oriented, to name a few possibilities. It can pertain in a larger sense to a public health campaign or it can relate to one individual's coping patterns. Human communication is a continuous and dynamic process, with the nurse and patient not only sharing and interpreting information, but also developing a relationship.

THEORETICAL BACKGROUND

Human communication is multidimensional. Watzlawick, Beavin, and Jackson (1967) believe that communication occurs on two levels: the relationship level and the content level. The relationship level refers to how the two participants are bound to each other. The content level refers to the words, language, and information. The two levels are inextricably bound. The content is relayed more effectively in healthy relationships. The opposite occurs in strained relationships; the message is not clearly relayed or heard because of struggles within the relationship.

Relationships between patients and health care providers influence communication and care. Communication has been studied in many disciplines involved in health care. The next section reviews three models of communication in the health-care setting, in order to provide a theoretical framework for communication. The models are:

- Health Belief Model
- King Interaction Model
- Therapeutic Model

The *Health Belief Model* (Rosenstock, 1974) focuses on the patient's perspective in health communication. This model has been influential because it tries to explain how the patient's beliefs can predict the adoption of healthy behaviors. Certain variables or modifying factors can influence a patient's beliefs. These include demographic characteristics like age, sex, and ethnicity; perceived threats; and cues to action (e.g., advice, advertising, or illness in a family member). For example, young adolescents are more susceptible to cigarette advertisements (cue to action) and peer pressure (age-related variable) than are middle-aged adults. The diagnosis of lung cancer in a family member (cue to action) would be more apt to influence a middle-aged adult to quit smoking than it would a teenager.

Communication in health care is influenced by the Health Belief Model. Cues to action are incorporated into interventions, to optimize their effectiveness in changing behaviors. Examples include advertising campaigns to stop adolescents from smoking and handouts for parents at the pediatrician's office encouraging childhood immunizations. Communication at the nurse-patient level should be geared toward understanding patients' perceptions of their health and utilizing interventions that are appropriate for their demographic characteristics and situational modifying factors.

The *King Interaction Model* (1971, 1981) emphasizes the communication process in the nurse-client relationship. The term *client* is used in this model. Interpersonal relationships in health care incorporate relationship, process, and transaction. The relationship between the nurse and the client begins with each making **judgments** about the other based on their **perceptions** of the situation. In the example, Mrs. T. feels that the nurse is forcing her to accept her medicines and scheduling without asking her opinion. The nurse perceives that Mrs. T. is having difficulty with the hospital schedule. These judgments lead to verbal and nonverbal **actions** that create reactions in both the client and the nurse. Mrs. T. feels frustrated by her inability to control the situation and is not communicating. The nurse, Jay, feels frustrated too because he does not understand Mrs. T.'s perceptions of the situation. The judgments, perceptions, actions, and reactions are all parts of the dynamic process of **interaction**. King describes **transactions** as the result of the shared communication and the relationship between the nurse and the client. Both participate in determining health-related goals. If Jay remains open and refrains from taking a defensive posture, he can relate Mrs. T.'s behavior and remarks to her lack of control in the hospital environment and fear about her diagnosis.

The *Therapeutic Model* describes the role of the relationship between the health care provider and the client. Carl Rogers (1951) described the therapeutic relationship as central to facilitating healthy adjustment in the client. Communication is client-centered because the patient is the focus of the interactions. The helper or health care provider communicates with empathy, positive regard (or respect), and congruence (or genuineness) to facilitate patient adjustment to the circumstances and movement toward health. In the example, the nurse can focus on Mrs. T.'s perceptions of the situation and offer suggestions about ways to incorporate her goals into the schedule. Although originally written for psychotherapists, *Rogerian Model* has proven useful for nursing and the establishment of the therapeutic nurse-patient relationship (see Chapter 5).

SUMMARY

Communication is the sharing of information between individuals. Communication is a dynamic process, as each person reacts to other participants involved in the relationship. The communication process is influenced by the content and the relationship. In health care communication, theoretical frameworks provide a basis for understanding the nurse-patient relationship.

The Health Belief Model is useful in understanding why patients adopt or change health behaviors. The King Interaction Model describes the nurse-patient relationship in terms of relationship, process, and transactions. The communication is influenced by perceptions and judgments made by both the patient and the nurse. The *Rogerian Model* describes a client-centered model for nurse-patient relationships. Nurses use empathy, congruence, and positive regard or respect to establish a therapeutic relationship with the patient. These selected models demonstrate the dynamic process of health care communication and the fundamental parts of the nurse-patient relationship.

CASE STUDY RESOLUTION

In the case study, Mrs. T. has certain perceptions about the nurse, Jay, and his behavior. Jay is unsure about her perceptions of him, his role, or her illness. What should have been a simple statement and intervention has become difficult because certain parts of communication are missing, and the relationship is not well-established. Perhaps Jay could respond, "Mrs. T., it is difficult to be a patient. You haven't had much time to yourself." Or "When would you like me to bring your medicine?" Or "You sound upset this morning." Whatever approach the nurse takes is essential to establishing mutual goals with this patient. The lack of communication, the perceptions on both sides, and the growing hostility in the patient and frustration in the nurse can minimize future communication and good nursing care.

EXERCISE

Break into groups of three. Each person in the group has a role: a nurse, a patient, and an observer. Each person in the group will role-play in one role for 5 minutes. Pick one of the scenarios. As the "nurse," begin the encounter with the appropriate introductions and assess the reason the "patient" has sought health care.

- A 17-year-old boy with a seizure disorder who is not taking medicines regularly.
- A 49-year-old man with a two-pack-a-day smoking habit for 35 years who has bronchitis.
- A 20-year-old woman with a chlamydial infection and a new sexual partner.
- A 77-year-old woman with a recent transient ischemic attack and dizziness who does not like using a cane.
- A 7-year-old boy who broke his wrist skateboarding and was not wearing protective gear.

As the "nurse," try to assess the "patient's" problem and arrive at mutually set goals. As the "observer," assess the "nurse's" actions using the following guidelines.

- Did the nurse begin the relationship with a warm, respectful manner?
- Did the nurse solicit the patient's perception of the situation?
- Did the nurse make judgments about the patient's behavior
- Was the nurse empathetic to the patient's feelings about the situation?
- Did the nurse ask the patient's opinion about possible interventions?
- Did the nurse incorporate the patient's health beliefs into the plan of care?

After each role-play, discuss your observations within your group.

Chapter *2*

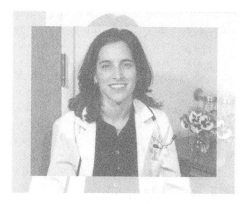

THE NURSE AS A PERSON

CASE STUDY

Susan is a 21-year-old senior in nursing school. She has always wanted to be a nurse but is having difficulty during the clinical rotation in pediatrics. For the past 2 clinical days, she has been assigned to work with Alyssa, a 4-year-old with acute lymphocytic leukemia. While undergoing maintenance chemotherapy, Alyssa has developed a fever of unknown origin. While Susan is changing Alyssa's pajamas, she looks at the little girl, who has complete alopecia from chemotherapy and is pale and limp. Susan finds herself starting to cry. Alyssa asks Susan, "What's wrong? Are you hurt?"

INTRODUCTION

Nurses, like all human beings, are complex organisms with feelings, fears, hopes, and needs. And, like other humans, nurses are the product of their genetic make-up, family environment, and cultural background. Becoming an effective nurse requires identifying the characteristics that make each person unique. The process of self-examination requires a more personal and honest reflection about the effect of past and present influences on current behavior. Most nursing students want to develop into kind, respectful, and effective professionals. They are motivated to understand and work with their patients to promote healing. However, a caring nurse requires working on understanding the variety of human responses to the stressful and challenging circumstances that often arise in the health care setting. Students need to develop into nurses who use the knowledge and skills of nursing in a manner that allows for accurate assessments, mutual goal setting, and timely interventions. Understanding human responses, both the nurse's and the patient's, requires knowledge of the self.

Self-Awareness

The terms self, self-concept, known self, and self-awareness are frequently used in human developmental theories. The **self** is a personal definition of oneself distinct from other people. The **self-concept** is the judgments and attitudes about the self. It explains behavior and provides a framework for decision making. The **known self** comprises that part of the self that is consciously acknowledged. When choices are made within the context of the known self, then self-identity and self-worth are affirmed. **Self-awareness** is the active process of learning about the components of the self.

Understanding the self allows the nurse to interact therapeutically with patients. Nurses provide a bridge for patients negotiating external events and personal reactions to their health and interventions. If the nurse can separate his or her personal reactions from the patient's responses, then more effective interactions can take place. The focus of the relationship becomes the patient's needs and responses, and not the nurse's. A deeper understanding of the self promotes growth in the nurse personally and enhances professional communication with patients.

Theoretical Background

Many theorists have tried to explain the origins of the self. Harry Stack Sullivan (1892-1949) wrote extensively on how the self develops. Sullivan, an American psychoanalyst, believed that the self or **self-system** emerges during infancy as the result of an interpersonal relationship with a significant other. He identified two prime motivating factors for behavior: the *need for satisfaction* and the *need for security*. During the first year of life, if the basic needs for food, water, warmth, and tenderness are met, then the infant feels secure and satisfied. If, on the other hand, certain basic needs are not met, then tensions such as anxiety and fear develop in the child. A lack of security during childhood can produce anxiety that stifles the development of healthy relationships in the adult.

On the professional level, Sullivan described the therapeutic relationship as a healing, human connection between the provider and the patient (see Chapter 5).

The nursing theorist Hildegard Peplau built on Sullivan's theories, applying them to nursing practice. Peplau (1952) defined nursing as a significant, therapeutic, and interpersonal process that functions cooperatively with other human processes to make health possible. She was the first to develop an interpersonal model of nursing practice, moving away from what nurses do **to** patients to what nurses do **with** patients. Nursing is not just a process of observation and intervention. Nurses actively engage with their patients in six roles, as defined by Peplau.

1. Stranger role—The nurse receives the patient as a stranger providing a climate that promotes trust.

2. Resource role—The nurse gives information, answers questions, and interprets clinical information.

3. Teaching role—The nurse serves as teacher to the learner/patient, giving instruction and training.

4. Counseling role—The nurse provides guidance and encouragement to help the patient integrate his or her current life experience.

5. Surrogate role—The nurse works on the patient's behalf and helps the patient clarify domains of independence, dependence, and interdependence.

6. Active leadership role—The nurse assists the patient in achieving responsibility for treatment goals in a mutually satisfying way.

Further development of Peplau's theory described the nurse-patient relationship as a dynamic process that creates the opportunity for learning and growth for both the patient and the nurse (1992). This working relationship has three phases, as described by Peplau:

- The orientation phase
- The working phase
- The resolution phase

During the orientation phase, the nurse and patient meet each other as strangers and develop a working partnership to address the health concerns of the patient. The nurse also performs an assessment of the patient's needs.

The working phase has two components: *identification* and *exploitation*. The identification component is when the nurse and patient clarify ideas and expectations for the relationship and the nurse develops a nursing care plan. During the exploitation part of the working phase, the nurse helps the patient identify health care services and personal resources and implement strategies to resolve the health issues.

During the resolution phase, the nurse and patient evaluate the current health status, and the nurse makes referrals, as necessary, to continue care beyond the relationship. (Further exploration of the nurse-patient relationship is in Chapter 5.)

Watson's *Theory of the Science of Caring*, first published in 1979, describes nursing interactions as "carative." The practice of caring is central to nursing and not just an emotion or a benevolent attitude. It is based on two human care values:

1. Care and love are the primal and universal psychic energy.
2. Care and love are necessary for our survival.

Theorists from other disciplines further developed the understanding of interpersonal communication. Sigmund Freud (1937) provided well-known insights into human behavior. Freud is famous for his descriptions of the id, ego, and superego, but he also developed the ideas of transference and countertransference. Transference is the projection of the one's attitudes or feelings from the past onto people in the present. For example, a female patient who is nervous about an upcoming surgery may say, "My husband hates hospitals." Countertransference refers to feelings that a nurse may develop about a patient's behaviors that have their roots in the nurse's previous life experiences. Take, for example, a nurse caring for a male patient who is angry about being hospitalized. Because of a negative childhood experience with anger in a male family member, the nurse avoids caring for the patient. Recognizing feelings of countertransference helps the nurse acknowledge her or his own feelings and allows a more objective reaction to the patient's responses. Often, sharing these confusing feelings with a colleague can help the nurse gain perspective about personality traits that inhibit responses or elicit negative or prejudiced judgments.

Freud also identified "ego defense mechanisms." These allow a person to protect himself or herself during anxiety-producing situations. Examples include denial, projection, and rationalization.

Denial is the lack of acceptance of a proven condition. For example, the mother whose child has leukemia cannot say that her child has cancer but she can acknowledge that her child requires chemotherapy.

Projection is the placing of one's own emotions onto another. For example, a nurse who is angry about her assignment tells her nurse manager that a colleague is upset about the heavy workload.

Rationalizations are used to justify ideas or feelings that feel illogical with seemingly reasonable explanations. For example, the patient with a 60-pack-a-year smoking history develops lung cancer. He explains that this happened because he used a wood stove to heat his house.

Nurses can also use these defense mechanisms to preserve their self-respect, reduce feelings of guilt, or maintain social acceptance with their peers.

Understanding how patients and nurses use these mechanisms to protect themselves allows for greater acceptance of the human responses to stressful circumstances and more evolved approaches to resolving maladaptive behaviors.

Carl Rogers (1961) explored the client-centered, or patient-centered, relationship and emphasized the healing powers of a successful, therapeutic relationship. He identified essential characteristics in the helper or nurse: genuineness and unconditional positive regard or respect.

Genuineness refers to the ability to be one's own self while being a professional. Responding to a comical remark with laughter, expressing condolences to a patient suffering loss, and being humble when at a loss for answers are examples of genuineness. Self-revelations make the nurse appear more human so the patient feels more comfortable revealing parts of himself or herself to the nurse.

Unconditional positive regard or respect is the ability to accept the patient's beliefs and attitudes despite the nurse's personal feelings about them. Patients have to adapt to their health and environment in their own ways, using strategies that have worked in the past. For example, a patient with a known substance abuse problem has now tested positive for human immunodeficiency virus (HIV). It might be frustrating to care for this patient. The nurse's job is to separate personal reactions from the situation. Interventions include helping the patient adapt, changing the high-risk behaviors, adopting health-preserving behaviors, and preventing further spread of the virus.

Erik Erikson (1902-1994) described the stages of personality development as a lifelong process (Table 2-1). The eight stages (Erikson, 1963) occur in a linear manner over time and can be influenced by social and environmental forces. The positive resolution of each stage allows for normal growth and development and passage into the next stage. Society reinforces the successful achievement of the stages with ceremonies like weddings, graduations, and retirement parties. Understanding these stages allows the nurse to understand where patients are developmentally.

As people mature, they develop more complex social skills. Life crises like the death of a loved one or a new illness might affect the mastery of particular developmental tasks. The passage to the next stage might be more difficult or arrested, or regression to a previous stage might occur. A child who experiences the divorce of his or her parents during muscular-anal stage may regress from being toilet-trained to having accidents. As he or she adapts to the changes in his or her life, the child will regain control and move to the next stage of development. The development of identity or self, is a central life process. Unexpected life circumstances like illness are threads in the tapestry of each person's life. Erikson's theory provides a view of life as a rich, unique fabric with expected patterns or stages but also with a variety of colors.

Table 2-1
Erikson's Stages of Personality Development

Age	Critical Task to be Accomplished	Qualities
Oral-sensory (0 to 2 years)	Trust vs. mistrust	To receive, to give
Muscular-anal (2 to 4 years)	Autonomy	To control, to let go
Locomotor-genital (4 to 6 years)	Initiative vs. guilt	To make, to play act
Latency (6 to 12 years)	Industry vs. inferiority	To make things, to put things together
Puberty and adolescence (13 to 19 years)	Identity vs. role confusion	To be one's self
Young adult	Intimacy vs. isolation	To share one's self with another
Adult	Generativity vs. stagnation	To take care of, to create
Maturity	Integrity vs. despair	To accept being, to accept not being

Abraham Maslow (1908-1970) was an American psychiatrist who developed a hierarchic categorization of human needs. The needs are stacked like a pyramid, with the most basic physiological needs (food, water, and air) at the base taking precedence over higher needs (love and belonging). If the first level of needs (physiologic needs) is met, then the second level of needs, for physical safety and security, can be achieved. Once the first two levels are met, humans need to feel love and belonging, such as to a family and/or community (love and belonging needs). People who feel a part of their community experience increased dignity, respect, and approval from others (self-esteem needs). The fifth or highest level of human needs is the level of self-actualization (Figure 2-1).

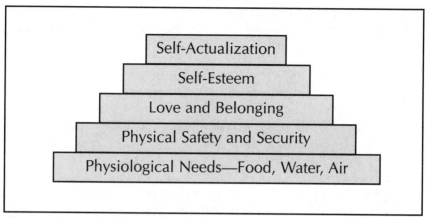

Figure 2-1. Maslow's hierarchy of human needs.

To become self-actualized, people must have met their needs at all the other levels. Then they can use their talents and personalities to the best of their abilities, for the betterment of society. Self-actualized people are not perfect or free from fears and worries. They use themselves openly, allowing others to view their strengths and weaknesses and using themselves to improve the lives of others. The qualities of a self-actualized person are:
- Full acceptance of self and others
- Integrity of purpose
- Quality of genuineness
- Ability to get along well with others
- Strong sense of personal worth
- "Peak experiences"—moments of intense emotional meaning
- Ability to view life experiences as opportunities, not threats
- Strong desire to serve humanity
- Identification with fellow human beings (Adapted from Arnold and Boggs, 1999)

Current developmental theorists look at the complexity of the self-concept. Travelbee (1971) describes the self-concept as unique to each person. Inborn personality traits, ethnic heritage, and physiologic characteristics are different for each person. Even family environment can be experienced differently by siblings. Life experiences are unique for each person, both quantitatively and qualitatively.

THE NURSE AS A PERSON

How do all these theories contribute to the development of a nurse? Understanding one's self as a person, the essence of self, is a lifelong goal, one that continues throughout a nurse's career and life. To paraphrase Carl Rogers (1961), people knowingly or unknowingly pursue this goal throughout life. To understand oneself allows fuller participation in life, as a nurse and as a human being. To recognize and accept oneself also allows fuller acceptance of others: their strengths and weaknesses, their loves and fears. When the nurse fully accepts others, he or she can experience true empathy, compassion, and caring.

Nurses come to the same profession from many different backgrounds. Many childhood experiences influence adult behavior. Relationships with our significant others play an important role in the development of self-identity.

One's view of the world begins with experiences within the family. Fawcett (1975) described the family as a living, open system. In *family systems theory*, the family is seen as a unified whole, constantly changing and reorganizing to adapt to information, energy, and matter from the surrounding environment. Every family has a unique pattern, shared values, and boundaries that separate the family from those outside the family system.

Family interactions develop over time, as individual family members react to each other. Bowen (1985) viewed the family as an emotional system in which each member has a role in maintaining family stability and reducing tension. Ways of communicating are passed from generation to generation, and, until a member challenges the system, the communication pattern and roles persist.

No one grew up in a perfect home or with perfect parents. While small children idolize their parents, adolescents give up these notions and begin to accept their parents as human beings. Even as adults, the memories of childhood tend to be idealized, but reviewing childhood experiences with adult eyes provides insight into one's reactions to life.

Communication styles differ between family systems. Healthy families provide a safe, secure environment where family members feel supported and valued. Members of healthy families care for each other, encouraging those in need, celebrating each other's accomplishments, and openly expressing emotions, while being considerate of others. Rules and values are clear, and a consistent hierarchy exists. Healthy communication allows for the expression of feelings and beliefs. Being a part of a healthy family means feeling supported in times of stress.

In troubled or unhealthy families, the adults might be a strictly authoritarian or unavailable parent—either physically or emotionally. They might avoid anger and confrontation, be openly hostile, or even physically violent. Questions from children are discouraged or considered "bad" behavior. Children repress their true feelings and natural curiosity so as not to upset the parents or elicit negative responses.

Unhealthy families can produce "early helpers": children who take on adult responsibilities while repressing their own needs and feelings. "Early helpers" may enter "helping" professions to meet a variety of their own conscious or unconscious needs: to receive affection, to control others, or to be depended upon. Children raised in unhealthy families may have feelings of low self-esteem, shame, and victimization. "Early helpers" are also at risk for substance abuse and addiction to comfort or numb the uncomfortable feelings, but they also have an amazing ability to cope and survive, to grow and be brave, in situations where others may not have the strength.

SUMMARY

Nurses come from a variety of families. Understanding yourself as a product of a family system allows for introspection and growth. Discovering oneself is a personal journey and a lifelong process. Feelings of self-worth, security, and autonomy must arise from a sense of self-awareness. Nurses as people need to take responsibility for their personal growth, acknowledging strengths and confronting negative feelings. Learning to be more sensitive and compassionate frees you from prejudice and negativity. Do not be afraid to look inside: discover goals and fears, loves and needs, strengths and weaknesses. They are present in all of us, creating uniqueness in each of us. Understanding yourself allows you to be an effective and caring provider, combining skill, knowledge, and compassion with your own unique personality.

CASE STUDY RESOLUTION

Susan was caught by surprise when Alyssa asked the question, "Are you hurt?" Susan responded, "No, I am not hurt. How are you feeling?" She held back her tears and finished caring for Alyssa. Afterwards, she sought out her instructor who, seeing her face, found a private place for them to talk. Susan talked about how hard it was to care for Alyssa. Susan has a niece about the same age as Alyssa and it made her think about Alyssa's illness. The instructor was supportive, telling Susan that sometimes situations with patients remind the nurse of personal relationships. Separating personal from professional feelings is an important and sometimes difficult part of being a nurse. Susan had developed a good relationship with Alyssa, making her comfortable and even making her laugh about the silly pictures she had drawn. Susan decided to continue caring for Alyssa that day. On Susan's return to the unit the following week, she learned that Alyssa's fever had resolved on antibiotics and she had been discharged.

Exercise 1

Complete the following statements honestly and confidentially. This exercise will help you look at some parts of yourself. It might take a week to complete this exercise, but take your time and see what you know (and don't know) about yourself. Afterwards, write a description of yourself. Who are you now? What do you like about yourself? What would you change? What personal qualities will make you a good nurse? What behaviors will you need to observe and change to be a more effective nurse?

- I would describe myself as...
- My family would describe me as...
- My friends think I am...
- I am proudest of...
- I get angry when...
- I am happy when...
- The characteristic I most like about myself is...
- Sometimes I get embarrassed when...
- The thing I want most to change about myself is...
- I get most nervous about...
- When I am under stress, I...
- I think that most people are...
- The characteristic I most dislike in others is...
- The best parts of my communication style are...
- The parts of my communication style that I need to improve are...
- My goal(s) for this course are...
- My goals for the next 5 years are...

Exercise 2

Break into groups of three. On a piece of paper, take 5 minutes to make a timeline of six major events in your life so far. Label each milestone according to Erickson's scheme. Then take 5 minutes to answer the following questions:

- Using the theorist Erik Erikson's scheme, what stage are you in?
- Looking at Maslow's hierarchy of needs, which of your needs are met and not met?
- Do you know someone who is self-actualized? Describe the qualities that this person possesses.

In your small groups, share your answer to only one of the questions. You can share your timeline or your description of a self-actualized person.

Now, share your responses with the entire group. Which are the most common milestones on the lifelines? Do certain milestones have overlapping stages in Erikson's scheme? What characteristics do the self-actualized people you described have in common?

Chapter 3

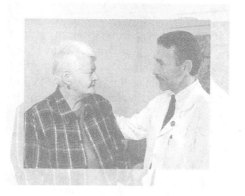

PATIENTS AS PEOPLE
Standards to Guide Communication

CASE STUDY

Mr. A. is a 67-year-old man with many physical problems. He has chronic obstructive pulmonary disease from an 80-pack-a-year smoking history. Plagued with arteriosclerosis, he recently had a stroke and a myocardial infarction. After his discharge from the hospital, the parish nurse has been visiting him in a skilled nursing facility. Despite his stroke, Mr. A. is very aware of the implications of his condition. The physician feels that his chances of returning home are slim and that his prognosis is very poor. In addition, his family has told him that he cannot smoke anymore and they will no longer bring him cigarettes. As the parish nurse is preparing to end a visit, she asks Mr. A. if there is anything she can do for him. He responds, "All I want is a cigarette. I know that I am never going to get out of this place. I have made my peace with God. I am ready to go. All I want is a cigarette. Could you bring me one?"

What would you do?

INTRODUCTION

When a patient and a nurse begin a relationship, a unique agreement takes place. The patient acknowledges your role as a nurse with the understanding that you have his or her best interests at heart. You will do what is right for this patient based on an understanding of patient rights, professional standards, ethical principles, and legal statutes. Your primary goal is always the health, well-being, and safety of the patient (American Nurses Association [ANA] Code of Ethics, 2002). The professional nurse combines these guiding determinants with the patient's values and beliefs, to mutually determine the goals of treatment.

PATIENT RIGHTS

Nursing has traditionally believed in the worth and dignity of all patients who require nursing care. The principle of self-determination or autonomy guides interventions. With roots in the ethical tradition of respect for persons, self-determination is the basis for informed decision making. Patients have the right to determine what will and will not be done to them in health care. Nurses help patients remain autonomous by providing information that is understandable to the patient, helping patients weigh the benefits and side effects of treatment, presenting all options, including withholding treatment, and supporting the patient in the decision-making process. Advance directives are an example of patient's making choices about care. A "do not resuscitate" order or a living will are examples of patients making choices about interventions prior to circumstances that could limit their ability to make their choices known. When a patient is unable to make decisions, a surrogate is designated to make decisions based on the patient's previously expressed wishes. Nurses should encourage their patients to review their rights and make decisions about potential interventions before a health crisis arises.

INSTITUTIONAL STANDARDS

During the 1960s, a movement emerged for patients' rights in health care. It arose in response to the public's desire to improve the quality of health care and make the system more responsive to the patients' needs. Patients wanted more control in determining their health care (the concept of self-determination). Today patients assume responsibility for their health and adopt preventative health care behaviors. Providers share in this responsibility when they educate the patient and the community about primary prevention and early detection. The provider and the patient share in the responsibility for determining the best care for each patient.

The American Hospital Association published "A Patient's Bill of Rights" in 1973 (and revised it in 1992). Its purpose is to promote the rights of the hospitalized patient. Hospitals have adopted this document and provide each patient with a printed copy. Some important parts include:

- The right to considerate and respectful care.
- The right to privacy, including confidentiality of all records of their care.
- The right to make decisions about their care, including the right to refuse care or treatment.
- The right to review all medical records and have them explained.
- The right to refuse to participate in research studies.
- The right to make statements about their care, including a living will and advance care directives.
- The right to be informed of resources in the hospital to resolve disputes or grievances.

While many of these rights may seem obvious, they were never formally adopted until the 1970s. Many insurance companies and health maintenance organizations also offer bills of rights. In these bills of rights, the same themes about patient care and communication keep reappearing: respect, confidentiality, and privacy. These are also the tenets of good communication and establishment of a therapeutic relationship.

PROFESSIONAL STANDARDS

Nurses, like other professions, require specific standards to define the scope of their knowledge and practice. The ANA has written the *Standards of Clinical Nursing Practice* and the *Code of Ethics for Nurses* to define what nurses do (1973, 1991, 2002). These important guidelines not only define the scope of nursing practice but are also the standards by which nurses are held accountable by the public. They are the basis for state Nurse Practice Acts, legal documents approved by each state's legislature that describe the scope of nursing practice. **Scope of practice** refers to legal parameters of nursing practice, including direct care (such as administration of medications), coordination of care with other disciplines, and delegating care to other personnel. Nursing practice is overseen by the Board of Nursing in each state.

LEGAL STANDARDS

The boundaries and expectations of the nursing profession are defined by law. Legal statutes serve to protect the public and set the standards for professional nursing care. The legal standard "a reasonable standard of care" is based in tort law. This standard is defined as care that a reasonably prudent nurse would provide in a similar situation. The reasonable standard of care is used as a benchmark in courts of law to judge criminal negligence. It holds a nurse accountable for his/her actions or failure to act. Criminal negligence by a nurse includes failing to protect a patient from harm, performing a nursing action that a reasonably prudent nurse would not perform, or failing to perform an action that a reasonably prudent nurse would perform. For example, if a nurse hears a patient talking about methods to kill himself and does nothing to protect the patient from himself, then this is criminally negligent behavior. Other examples of unprofessional conduct include breaching patient confidentiality, performing actions without sufficient preparation, failure to report or document changes in a patient's status, verbally or physically abusing a patient, and falsifying records.

Confidentiality

Patient confidentiality is an important issue from a professional, legal, and institutional point of view. Confidentiality stems from the ethical tradition of a right to privacy. Breaching a patient's confidential communication is a breach of trust and violates standards established by institutions and the government. New standards from the Office of Civil Rights/Health Insurance Portability and Accountability Act of 1996 (OCR/HIPPA) define the protection of patients' individually identifiable data arising from encounters with health care services. Only information that is pertinent to the patient's treatment is shared with other health care providers. Only those providers who have a "need to know" are given specific information. For example, if a worker sustained a back injury on the job, then only health information related to the injury would be given to the insurer regarding workers' compensation, not the entire medical record.

Legally, communication between a nurse and patient is considered **privileged communication**, and the nurse is forbidden by law from disclosing this information, with one exception. If this communication includes evidence that could harm innocent people including the patient himself or herself, then, legally and morally, this information must be shared with the appropriate authorities. Included in this exception are instances of child abuse, gunshot wounds, and communicable diseases.

Communication and Malpractice

Within the realm of legal issues pertaining to nursing practice lies the issue of malpractice. While it might be difficult to understand why a book on talking with patients would address this issue, good communication may be the best prevention against malpractice. Even though you work within the scope of nursing practice and maintain excellent clinical skills, you still might encounter the patient who is angry and feels the need to sue his or her health care providers. You might actually be named in a lawsuit, despite providing the best nursing care. On the other hand, patients who feel that they were treated with respect and compassion rarely sue. Patients who feel that their providers really listen to them are usually satisfied patients. Good "bedside manner" is not just secondary to being a nurse, it is essential to good nursing practice and patient satisfaction. So the same basic ideas—respect, empathy, and genuineness—can also prevent malpractice claims.

Communication Skills to Prevent Malpractice Claims

- Be respectful and genuine.
- Listen to what the patient says and doesn't say. Strive to understand his or her experience.
- Be available and accessible to the patient.
- Avoid rote phrases that demean what the patient feels.
- Be clear about the reasoning you use to reach decisions regarding the patient's care.
- Involve the patient in the informed consent process.
- Carry through with your commitments and do not make promises that you cannot keep.
- Be honest about what you know and do not know.

ETHICAL STANDARDS AND PRINCIPLES

Ethical resources serve to guide your decision making in the nurse-patient relationship. In order to establish any profession, a group must formulate and adhere to an ethical code. The nursing profession, through the ANA, developed *The Code of Ethics for Nurses* (1976, 1985; 2002) to express the expectations of ethical nursing practice and acknowledge the responsibility entrusted in the nursing profession by the public. The *Code* is:

- The nurse, in all professional relationships, practices with compassion and respect for the inherent dignity, worth, and uniqueness of every individual, unrestricted by considerations of social or economic status, personal attributes, or the nature of health problems.
- The nurse's primary commitment is to the patient, whether an individual, family, group, or community.
- The nurse promotes, advocates for, and strives to protect the health, safety, and rights of the patient.
- The nurse is responsible and accountable for individual nursing practice and determines the appropriate delegation of tasks consistent with the nurse's obligation to provide optimum patient care.
- The nurse owes the same duties to self as to others, including the responsibility to preserve integrity and safety, to maintain competence, and to continue personal and professional growth.

- The nurse participates in establishing, maintaining, and improving health care environments and conditions of employment conducive to the provision of quality health care and consistent with the values of the profession through individual and collective action.
- The nurse participates in the advancement of the profession through contributions to practice, education, administration, and knowledge development.
- The nurse collaborates with other health professionals and the public in promoting community, national, and international efforts to meet health needs.
- The profession of nursing as represented by associations and their members is responsible for articulating nursing values, for maintaining the integrity of the profession and its practice, and for shaping public policy.

Again, the same themes emerge to guide nursing interventions: respect and nonjudgmental care for every patient. The Code is a published and, therefore, public document of nursing practice that should drive and guide all nursing care. The Code is also the public's expectation of the services provided by a professional nurse.

The words **health care consumer, client, and patient** and are often used preferentially in articles and books. A health care consumer is one who purchases services from a health care provider. *Merriam-Webster's Collegiate Dictionary* (1996) provides definitions:

- Client—One who is under the protection of another, or a person who engages the professional advice or services of another.
- Patient—An individual awaiting or under medical care or treatment, or one that is acted upon, derived from "one who suffers."

Because the patient is in a vulnerable position that requires a level of trust and vigilance from the health care provider, the word **patient** is used in this book. Sometimes a patient is unconscious, anesthetized, or medicated, requiring nurses and other health care providers to make decisions with the family in the patient's best interest. The patient cannot choose or monitor the care he or she receives while in a compromised state. He or she must trust that his or her health care providers will intervene on his or her behalf. With a conscious patient, choices must be presented in a way that the patient can understand. Then, the nurse is often called upon to help the patient and his or her family with the decision-making process. This heavy responsibility brings with it moral and ethical obligations. While acknowledging that patients are also protected, the word *patient* is used in this book to symbolize the active and sometimes passive roles that patients assume during a health care experience. Health care providers are morally obliged to make decisions about their care with their best interests at heart.

VALUES

Moral reasoning and decision making require the ability to identify values: the nurse's values and the patient's values. As discussed in Chapter 2, the nurse brings a set of values to the professional role. Some values come from one's cultural and ethnic background. (See Chapter 4 for more on cultural diversity.) Others are based on personal experiences, beliefs, and attitudes. Throughout life, values are acquired from family, friends, religious groups, and community. It is important that the nurse delivers care in a manner that respects the patient's values and needs. It is also vital that the nurse identifies and respects the patient's values even if they differ from his or her own.

Values are a person's beliefs about the truth, beauty, and worth of any thought, object, or behavior. They give direction and meaning to life and guide the decision-making process. Values also determine behavior by guiding the responses to experiences and choices in life. You need to be aware and conscious of the values that influence behaviors and perceptions, respecting the patient's viewpoint and ability to make choices about his or her health care. Self-awareness will free you to focus on the patient's needs, and that freedom generates open communication.

ETHICAL DECISION MAKING

Helping patients to arrive at decisions about their care is fundamental to the nurse's role. Decision making is guided by the patient's values and beliefs. The nurse helps the patient to identify his or her values, potential conflicts, and goals. Self-awareness on the part of the nurse allows the patient's goals to be the focus of decision making. Often, difficult decisions bring emotional content to the process. The nurse works to support the patient's rights and integrity by interpreting the information are helping the patient to prioritize and make choices.

Steps in Ethical Decision Making

- Gather background information—Known information about the patient and the context of the situation.
- Identify ethical components—Underlying issues and who is affected.
- Clarify roles—Rights and obligations of all involved.
- Explore options—Alternatives, potential negative effects, goals, desired outcome.
- Apply ethical principles—Consider ethical theories, scientific facts.
- Resolve the dilemma—Consider the effects of the decision and implementation and how it will be evaluated (Stuart & Sundeen, 1991).

SPIRITUALITY

Spirituality, from the Latin word *spiritus* or breath, is an important aspect of every human being. It deals with a person's pursuit of meaning in life. It influences decisions and values. The spiritual dimension is such an integral part of each person that it influences responses to health and illness. Often this aspect of our humanness is overlooked in nursing because of more pressing patient needs or because of the nurse's discomfort with the subject.

Spirituality is different from religion. Spirituality includes a broader scope than religion. Religion tends to refer to an organized group and a codified set of beliefs and practices. Spirituality is a person's need for meaning and purpose in life, his or her need to love and be loved, and his/her need for hope and creativity (Highfield & Carson, 1983). The definition of spirituality often includes the person's relationship with a God or higher being or a concept of deity.

Health and spirituality are intricately linked. A patient's spiritual and/or religious background influences his/her values and beliefs, communication, and decision making. Patients may openly talk about their religious beliefs, but frequently this area remains underassessed. Holistic nursing care and optimum communication about health care decisions require an understanding of the patient's spiritual dimension. FICA is a quick Spiritual Assessment Tool (Pulcjaski & Romer, 2000) that can be used to start the discussion.

- Faith and beliefs—"What were you raised to believe?"
- Importance—"What role does religion play in your life?"
- Community—"Where do you practice your religion?"
- Address—"How can we meet your spiritual needs here?"

SUMMARY

People enter a health care setting with their own rights and values. Institutions, professions, and the government try to protect the rights of the person as a patient. In the profession of nursing, guidelines for practice are published by state and national nursing organizations. The goal of all guidelines, ethical principles, and legal statutes is to protect the patient. Incorporating professional guidelines with the patient's own values allows for nursing care that is unique and effective for each patient.

CASE STUDY RESOLUTION

The parish nurse thought through her beliefs about smoking and health, her relationship with Mr. A., and his prognosis. His health condition was very poor, and his future life was limited. It would bring him pleasure to have a cigarette and probably would not change his prognosis. Focusing on compassionate care and respect for this patient as a person, the parish nurse decided to bring Mr. A. a pack of cigarettes. He was very grateful and asked the nurse to roll his wheelchair outside so he could smoke. In the spring air, they talked about his life and what had made him happy. Mr. A. died 4 weeks later as the result of a urinary tract infection and renal failure.

EXERCISE

Value Priority Exercise

This exercise is aimed at increasing self-awareness and clarifying values. Read through the list of values and rate their level of importance to you:
1. Very important
2. Important
3. Not important

After completion, pick out the five highest rated values and the five with the lowest scores. Remember, there is no right or wrong answer. Try to be honest with yourself. This exercise is for your insight only.

Values:
- Achievement (accomplishment)
- Aesthetics (appreciation of beauty in art and nature)
- Altruism (service to others, interest in the well-being of others)
- Autonomy (personal freedom, self-determination)
- Creativity (developing new ideas)
- Emotional well-being (peace of mind, inner security)
- Health (physical and mental well-being)
- Honesty (being truthful and genuine)
- Justice (treating others fairly)
- Knowledge (pursuit of information, truth, principles)
- Love (caring, unselfish devotion)
- Loyalty (allegiance to a person or group)
- Morality (honor, integrity, keeping ethical standards)
- Physical appearance (concern for one's appearance, being well-groomed)
- Pleasure (fun, joy, gratification, enjoying life)
- Power (control, authority, influence over others)
- Recognition (being important, well-liked)
- Spirituality (having a religious belief)
- Wealth (having possessions or enough money)
- Wisdom (mature understanding, insight, good judgment)

Five Most Important Values:
1.
2.
3.
4.
5.

Five Least Important Values:
1.
2.
3.
4.
5.

Chapter 4

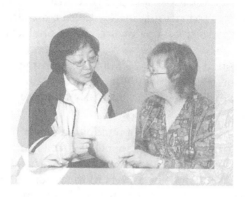

CULTURAL DIVERSITY
Translating Awareness into Competence

CASE STUDY

Mrs. C. is a 64-year-old woman who emigrated from China to America as a newlywed 40 years ago. Now she is scheduled to undergo a hysterectomy. The nurse in the surgeon's office is doing a preoperative assessment and teaching session with Mrs. C. Although Mrs. C. speaks and understands English well, she makes little direct eye contact and has no questions. She refuses the prescriptions for pain medicine. The nurse is about to obtain informed consent for the procedure, but is not sure that Mrs. C. understands what has been discussed. How would cultural awareness help in this situation?

INTRODUCTION

The health care workplace is a multicultural environment that requires special communication skills. There are many definitions of culture, some anthropological and some more behavior based. The word **culture** refers to the common beliefs, symbols, behaviors, and traditions that are passed from one generation to the next. Trying to define or describe a culture helps others to understand the experience of a particular group. Different cultures provide the diversity that makes America so rich in traditions. According to the United States Census data (2000), 25% of the population is composed of ethnic minorities. Nurses can expect to care for patients from different cultural backgrounds, with beliefs and values that may influence their responses and health behaviors.

Diversity refers to the existence of multiple cultures within the population of a country or a group. Diversity also includes factors other than ethnic origin, like gender, economic status, educational background, and sexual orientation. Patients arrive with many aspects to their cultural background, all of which affect their approach to life and health. To communicate in a way that is culturally competent requires an understanding that each patient is first of all an individual and second a part of one or more cultural groups.

Cultural awareness or **competence** is included in the educational standards of many health care professions. But what is cultural competence? Is it a viewpoint that increases awareness and respect for patients from cultures different from our own? Or is it the recognition that each person, including the nurse, is the product of our own cultural background?

THEORETICAL BACKGROUND

Leninger's Transcultural Care Theory was first published in 1978. She describes culture and caring as intricately linked. There can be no cure without caring, and caring values and behaviors differ between cultures. The goal of transcultural nursing is to develop a body of knowledge to provide culture-specific and culture-universal nursing interventions.

Bonder, Martin, and Miracle (2002) suggest that cultural competence can be learned by an **inquiry-centered** approach. By creating a particular mindset, health care providers can learn to generate hypotheses based on previous experiences with a cultural group. But the seasoned practitioner also knows when to generalize and when to individualize care. Cultural backgrounds are multi-faceted and individual. The hypotheses provide a foundation from which each patient is assessed as a unique person.

OBSTACLES TO CULTURAL AWARENESS

Two points need to be made about obstacles to cultural awareness. First, **ethnocentrism**, or the belief in the superiority of one's own ethnic group, is a major obstacle to effective communication. Although it is a universal tendency, ethnocentrism is dangerous because it not only blocks understanding, but it also can lead to prejudice against other cultural groups. **Prejudice** can be described as making judgments about others based on previous experiences. For example, if a patient like Mrs. C. comes from a culture where direct eye contact is considered disrespectful, and the nurse comes from a culture that views lack of direct eye contact as inattentive or insincere, then communication will be strained. To be effective, you need to try seeing from the patient's viewpoint, understanding that the patient's cultural background affects his or her communication and behavior.

The second obstacle to culturally competent communication is **stereotyping**. Given the rich ethnic and cultural traditions of the American population, the chances are that each patient embraces more than one set of beliefs and traditions. Nurses need to examine and acknowledge their personal assumptions about groups different from their own. Understanding the complexity of social, cultural, and economic factors allows the nurse to provide culturally sensitive and individualized care.

CULTURAL CHARACTERISTICS

Consideration of the different characteristics of culture helps to explain how communication varies among people, families, and communities. The two characteristics that are most commonly discussed are context and individual vs collective values. **Context** refers to the ways in which messages are interpreted. In high-context cultures, communication is interpreted by a set of culturally based rules. The status of the speaker and the nonverbal rules of communication are clearly established. For example, in the Japanese and Arab cultures, if a person of higher status is speaking (like the nurse or doctor), then the patient acquiesces to their recommendations. In low-context cultures, the focus is on the content of the message, with less attention to the status of the speaker. There are fewer nonverbal rules, and the meaning is the actual content of the message. American and German cultures are good examples of low-context cultures. Although there is a continuum for cultural context, it is helpful for nurses to understand that patients from high-context cultures usually speak less and are more attentive to nonverbal cues. Like in the example of Mrs. C., it might take more time to clarify her understanding of the surgery by using open-ended questions like, "How long will you avoid heavy lifting after your surgery?" Validation of the patient's beliefs can be incorporated into the teaching. For example, "Mrs. C., most patients experience pain after this surgery. The pain medicine will make it easier for you to move and breathe deeply. It will make your recovery easier." Implications for nursing care for patients from low-context cultures include providing pamphlets and handouts, because the actual sources of information are considered valuable.

The focus of the culture is a defining characteristic that can clarify intercultural communication. **Individualistic** cultures focus on the individual and their needs. Individualism stresses autonomous decision making. Independence is valued and people take care of themselves and their immediate families. Examples of individualistic cultures include the United States and Western European countries.

Collectivistic cultures focus on the needs of the group or community. Decisions are made with the consensus of the group. Harmony within the group is valued. Communication follows the rules of the group and attention is paid to authority. Collectivistic cultures include Asian-Pacific Islanders like Japanese and Pakistanis.

Understanding general cultural characteristics can improve intercultural communication and generate some basic ideas about culturally based beliefs. Although no one rule can apply to communication with all patients from one country or group, certain general cultural hypotheses can be drawn that use an inquiry-based approach to cultural assessment

How to Communicate Transculturally

- Consider the individual first and the cultural background second.
- Assess language needs and, if required, arrange for an interpreter or family member to translate.
- Approach the patient slowly and greet him or her respectfully, pronouncing his or her name correctly or asking how to pronounce the name.
- Do not raise your voice to be understood.
- Allow sufficient time and a quiet setting.
- Sit at the patient's level at a comfortable distance away from the patient.
- Listen to the patient's words and watch his or her nonverbal language.
- Reassure the patient that you are there to help and that any information he or she provides will be kept private.
- Try to mirror the patient's style of communicating (e.g., slow, quiet speech and little direct eye contact with Asian-Americans).
- Provide written material in the patient's language, if available.
- Allow time for questions.

Summary

First, you, as a nurse, need to try understanding your patient's perspective. Assess any basic hypotheses about a patient's cultural background with that individual. Second, assess and understand each patient as part of a family and cultural group(s) to improve your ability to develop a working, respectful relationship with the patient. Your patient is the "cultural informant" who shares his or her beliefs with you (DeSantis, 1994). Although a particular cultural group might hold certain beliefs, each patient responds differently to each circumstance. It is your role to assess each patient as a unique individual with a unique perspective. Then, you can integrate culturally specific interventions into the nursing care plan. Approach every patient with the knowledge that identity is the result of many complex factors and that each person can have many cultural identities.

CASE STUDY RESOLUTION

Mrs. C has a multicultural background. Although she has lived in America for a long time, she also has roots in Chinese culture. A collectivistic culture, Chinese people value the good of the community. Many also feel that the expression of pain is a sign of weakness. Too much eye contact may be viewed as disrespectful of authority figures. The nurse thinks about Mrs. C.'s cultural roots when continuing with the preoperative teaching. First, she asks Mrs. C. if she understands the surgery. Mrs. C. looks down and then at the nurse and says, "Of course I know that I need a hysterectomy. You have explained it all to me." She signs the informed consent. Then, the nurse reviews the need for pain medicine by almost all patients after a hysterectomy as beneficial for movement and deep breathing which will speed recovery and prevent some complications. It is routinely used. Mrs. C. reluctantly agrees that she may need pain medicine immediately after surgery. Mrs. C.'s surgery went well and she required little postoperative pain medication. She was discharged home in 3 days.

EXERCISE

Take a piece of paper and answer the following questions:
- What cultural backgrounds do you come from?
- What language is spoken in your family, your parents' families, your grandparents' families?
- What religions are parts of your family's traditions?
- Who makes the decisions in the family?
- How are the elderly viewed in your family?

In groups of five, share your answers and think about the following questions:
- Are people influenced by more than one culture?
- How many in the group have multiple ethnic backgrounds?
- How would the group define culture? Write a definition in one sentence.

Return to the whole group and share each small group's definition of culture.
- How are the definitions the same?
- Do the definitions include economic and educational background?
- How do social organization and power fit into the concept of culture?
- Does culture affect decision making?

The Nurse-Patient Relationship

Section 2

Chapter 5

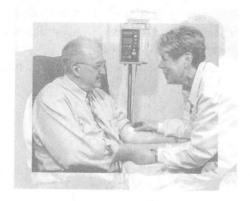

ESTABLISHING A THERAPEUTIC RELATIONSHIP

CASE STUDY

Susan R. is a 38-year-old woman coming into the outpatient surgery center for a breast biopsy. She sits in the waiting room with her husband and is obviously nervous: staring unblinking at the wall, tapping her feet, and wringing a tissue in her hand. The perioperative nurse approaches Susan to introduce herself and bring Susan back to prepare for surgery.

Nurse: "Mrs. R., I am Laurie Snow, and I will be the nurse caring for you today. What do you like to be called?"

Patient: "Hello. Call me Sue; that's what everyone else calls me. This is my husband, Rick."

Nurse: (She shakes hands with the patient and her husband.) "It's nice to meet both of you. Sue, I would like to explain what's going to happen today, ask you a few questions, and answer any questions that you may have about your surgery."

Patient: "Oh, thank you. I am so scared. I don't know how I am going to get through this."

Nurse: "You are nervous about the surgery. My goal is to help you through today. I will explain everything as we go along."

Patient: "I am glad that you will be there. May my husband come with me?"

Nurse: "Of course."

INTRODUCTION

In a few moments, this nurse has accomplished a great deal toward making a strong nurse-patient relationship. What did she do?
- She identified herself by name.
- She established her credentials and her role.
- She acknowledged the patient by her preferred name.
- She respectfully addressed both the patient and her husband.
- She reflected the patient's response to the surgery.
- She offered her assistance in relieving the patient's anxiety by explaining her role.
- She acknowledged that the patient has questions that might be contributing to her anxiety.

Good communication skills make the difference. The therapeutic relationship forms the basis of nursing care for the patient and the patient's family throughout the spectrum of health and illness. Some relationships like the one in this example only last a few hours, but others may last days, months, or years. What is exciting about each relationship is how unique and enriching it can be. The underlying principles in the therapeutic relationship are the same regardless of the length of the contact: respect, genuineness, empathy, active listening, trust, and confidentiality. A therapeutic relationship is different from a social relationship because it is health-focused and patient-centered with defined boundaries. Peplau (1991) described this one-way interest as "professional closeness." The purpose of the therapeutic relationship is to support the patient, to promote healing, and to support or enhance functioning.

Communication in the nurse-patient relationship focuses on the patient's needs, taking into consideration multiple factors. The nurse must contemplate the patient's physical and emotional condition, cultural background, readiness to communicate, and ways of relating to others. For example, talking about a low cholesterol diet is not appropriate during the acute phase of a myocardial infarction. The patient is not in the correct physical or emotional state. Later, when the patient is preparing to be discharged, teaching about health-promoting behaviors like diet and exercise is appropriate.

RESPECT (UNCONDITIONAL POSITIVE REGARD)

Carl Rogers defined respect or unconditional positive regard as the ability to accept another person's beliefs and responses despite your own personal feelings. Each patient's response to health or illness is a personal way of adapting to the circumstances (see Chapter 3). Each patient brings a lifetime of responding and coping to the challenges of life. The nurse needs to be nonjudgmental regarding these responses and seek to respect the patient as a human being. Acceptance does not mean approval or agreement. It is a nonjudgmental attitude about the patient as a whole person. The goal is to make the patient feel comfortable and legitimize his or her feelings. For example, the nurse might not always understand why patients become angry, but acknowledges that they usually have reasons, based on their beliefs and backgrounds, for feeling that way. Some patients might have habits, like smoking or excessive drinking, that they will not change despite the nurse's best efforts at teaching health-promoting behaviors. Some patients might have difficulty maintaining personal hygiene. The nurse's goal is to respectfully take into account the patient's symptoms, feelings, values, and beliefs and work with the patient to plan the goals for treatment.

How to Show Respect

- Introduce yourself by name and professional status and wear a name tag.
- Ask your patient what he or she likes to be called. Always begin with the formal (e.g., Mr., Ms., Mrs.), and then address the patient by his or her preferred name.
- Arrange for patient comfort and privacy.
- Warn the patient before doing any procedures, particularly those that involve personal space or discomfort.
- Respond to your patient in ways that demonstrate that you understand what he or she has said.

GENUINENESS

The ability to be oneself within a professional role is called **genuineness**. Rogers described genuineness as congruence, but the meaning is the same: to have the professional self in agreement with the personal self. This is not always easy because, out of respect to patients, the nurse cannot make judgments about their values. However, if the nurse truly cares about the patient, then his or her personality and caring will show through within and beyond the bounds of professional behavior. Genuineness is a welcome part of the health care experience, because it allows a sharing of the human parts of life.

Patient: "I have some bad news. I started smoking again. I tried, really tried, but everyone at home was smoking."

Nurse: "I am glad that you tried to quit. It's tough, isn't it? Many people try to quit three or even five times before succeeding. If you stop smoking, you will help your chronic bronchitis. Let's talk about other strategies for quitting smoking. Where can your family smoke that is away from you?"

In this short interchange, the nurse acknowledged the patient's efforts and the difficulties in his life, offered encouragement, and started working with the patient to solve the problem.

Another way you can be genuine is to allow interest in the patient as a person to show during daily nursing care. As time allows, ask about the patient's family, work, hobbies, or ability to carry out his or her normal routine. Older patients enjoy sharing life experiences. This is not just superficial chatter. This information allows you to understand the patient's life, priorities, and coping patterns during a change in health status. Encouraging patients to share their life stories shows an interest in them as people and not just as a diagnosis or procedure.

Genuineness, even as a student nurse, is freeing. The first time a student experiences a conflict in congruence might be when introducing himself or herself as a student to a patient. Although it might feel difficult, a student nurse should introduce himself or herself as a student, reaffirming that although his or her knowledge is limited, the interest in the patient is not. Even as a practicing nurse, there will be times when time, knowledge, or ability will be limited, and that sincere revelation to the patient does not make a "bad" nurse, but an honest one.

Nurses can genuinely express other feelings within the therapeutic relationship. For example, you can laugh when a patient brings in a joke from the Internet that is appropriate and funny. Likewise, you can express sympathy to the patient who has recently lost a loved one.

SELF-DISCLOSURE

Self-disclosure is a tricky topic for many students and nurses. They want to appear professional and not divulge personal details or feelings. Professors encourage students to keep the focus of the interactions on the patient. The reality of the therapeutic relationship might be different, and students are at a loss to define personal and professional boundaries. Spontaneous questions and sharing do occur during interactions with patients. But what is appropriate? Patients might ask questions about personal details like, "Where are you from?" or "Do you have any children?" These questions might be used by the patient to find common ground for conversation or to make them more comfortable about their revelation of personal details. Whatever the reason, the student and professional nurse needs to establish, first, that the patient is the focus of the time together. Then, as time or the relationship permits, the sharing of other information may be appropriate. Intimate details are never shared by the nurse. When in doubt, the nurse should ask another trusted colleague or professor about a particular question. It is always within the nurse's bounds to say, "I don't think that question is relevant to your care. Let's focus on you..."

EMPATHY

Empathy is understanding the experience of another. It is not sympathy or pity. **Sympathy** is actually experiencing what the patient is feeling. **Pity** is feeling sorry for someone. Empathy, on the other hand, is the ability to understand what a patient is experiencing from his or her perspective. Sympathy can impair the nurse's ability to make objective judgments in a realistic manner, because emotion might cloud the issues. Empathy is the ability to actually see the world from another's point of view without experiencing the emotional content.

Empathy is a form of understanding and participation in the patient's world. It is important to understand how the patient responds both physically and emotionally to his or her experience. Empathy allows the nurse to focus on the patient's needs. Interventions are focused on the individual patient's health issues and also on his or her abilities to cope and adapt to changes in functioning. The empathetic nurse understands the patient's experience, sets goals with the patient, and customizes the interventions to meet these goals.

TRUST

Establishing trust is vitally important to therapeutic communication. Trust is the foundation of all interpersonal relationships. The development of a sense of trust is a primal need in psychoanalytic theories (see Chapter 2), but it is essential when a patient is placed in a vulnerable position, physically and emotionally. The patient needs to believe that the nurse is honest, dependable, and accepting of who they are. Erikson (1963) described trust as the reliance on consistency, sameness, and continuity of experiences provided by familiar and predictable things and people. Trust is a choice that people make, based on their need to trust others. Nurses can facilitate the process of developing trust with certain behaviors.

Facilitating Trust

- Listen carefully, and your patient will feel that you understand and care.
- Treat your patient respectfully, and he or she will feel like a valued human being.

- Be honest and consistent, and your patient will feel that you are trust-worthy.
- Follow through on your commitments, and your patient will feel that your care is predictable and dependable.
- Have an accepting attitude, and your patient will be more comfortable sharing parts of himself or herself.

CONFIDENTIALITY

Moral principles dictate the practice of nursing. The nurse has moral and legal obligations not to share patient information with others, except in specific circumstances. It is important from the standpoint of trust that patients know that their personal information will be kept confidential, even if they do not request it. This includes taking care not to speak in public places or where information could be overheard, like elevators and cafeterias. It also includes confidentiality with electronic information. Care should be taken to arrange for privacy in the physical setting before discussing sensitive information. Providing privacy may include finding an empty room or asking an ambulatory roommate to leave or closing the door to a patient's room. The only reasons that nurse-patient confidentiality can be breached are:
- Suspicion of abuse of minors or elders
- Commission of a crime
- Threat of harm to oneself or others

(For more on confidentiality, see Chapter 3)

THE NURSE-PATIENT RELATIONSHIP

The establishment of the nurse-patient relationship is a conscious commitment on the part of the nurse to care for a patient. The nurse accepts primary responsibility for setting the structure and purpose of the relationship. Using the concepts of respect, empathy, trust, genuineness, active listening, and confidentiality, the nurse begins to establish rapport with the patient and the family. The nurse functions within professional, legal, ethical, and personal boundaries (see Chapter 2). The nurse also appreciates the uniqueness of each patient and strives to understand his or her response to changes in health.

Hildegard Peplau, the nursing theorist, identified four phases of the nurse-patient relationship: orientation, identification, exploitation, and resolution. The phases are therapeutic and focus on interpersonal therapeutic interactions.
1. Orientation—The patient seeks help, and the nurse assists the patient to identify the problem and the extent of help needed.

2. Identification—The patient relates to the nurse from an independent, dependent, or interdependent posture, and the nurse assures the patient that he or she understands the meaning of his or her situation.

3. Exploitation—The patient uses the nurse's services and other resources on the basis of his or her needs.

4. Resolution—The patient's old needs are resolved, and more mature goals emerge.

Orientation Phase

Beginning the nurse-patient relationship requires unique communication skills. Every day people communicate with those around them by listening, talking, sharing, laughing, reassuring, and caring. Nurses use these basic components of communication to establish a helping relationship. Although different from the other relationships in life like friendships, family roles, casual contacts, and professional alliances, the relationship between a nurse and a patient is still a connection between people. Particular communication skills are effective to begin this unique relationship with a patient.

During the **orientation phase**, the relationship formally begins. The nurse sets the tone for the relationship by greeting the patient properly. "I am Laurie Snow and I will be the nurse taking care of you during the day today." The nurse introduces herself by name and professional status with a handshake and a smile. The tone and warmth of the words can promote connectedness between the nurse and the patient. The patient is called by the formal name first and then asked what he or she prefers to be called. Establishing rapport might begin with talking about neutral topics like the patient's hobbies and interests. This shows the patient that the nurse is interested in the patient as a person. Trust is also developed during this phase. The nurse can foster trust by being dependable and consistent in his or her actions. Through words and actions, the nurse conveys warmth and competence. This first phase is important in developing a foundation for the therapeutic relationship.

After the greeting phase, the nurse clarifies the purpose and nature of the relationship. This includes information about the appointment or interview, description of the nurse's role, helping the patient provide pertinent information, and describing the goals of the relationship. Each nurse has a personal style, and the delivery of this information will vary. What is important is not overlooking this part of the relationship. Establishing the purpose and goals of the relationship is fundamental not only to the delivery of care but also to the evaluation of the relationship during the termination phase. Also, anxiety levels decrease when the patient knows what to expect and participates in the establishment of the relationship. The nurse seeks to promote trust and reduce anxiety by being genuine and respectful. Receptive body language, active listening, and consistency help the patient feel more comfortable and be more focused.

Data collection occurs during the orientation phase. The nursing assessment serves as a guide for collecting relevant information from the patient about his or her health status and functioning. The nurse needs an open mind to understand the patient's perception of the problem and the need for treatment. What might seem apparent to the nurse might not be the patient's view of the situation. For example, the nurse could begin with a general question, "What brought you into the hospital today?" or "What kind of assistance can we provide for you?" While more specific questions on the nursing assessment might provide a focus for the initial data collection, it is important for the nurse to take the time to listen—really hear—the patient's needs and expectations. This prevents disappointment during and at the end of the relationship, if care did not proceed as the patient anticipated. The nurse can correct misinformation and clarify the situation.

The orientation phase ends with a therapeutic contract. While not always a formal document, the contract explains the roles of the nurse and patient and the goals of the relationship. From the earlier case study, the nurse concludes the initial meeting with the patient, by saying, "Sue, I will be with you throughout your breast biopsy, now through when you go home. I will start with a brief questionnaire. Then, I will explain what will happen today. Do you have any other questions at this time?"

Identification Phase

The working segment of the relationship begins with the **identification phase**. The nurse and patient work together to identify problems and set specific problem-oriented goals. Health problems are identified during data collection and appropriate interventions are developed in the nursing care plan. Mutual goal setting allows the patient to feel he or she is an active participant in his or her care. Nurses can also help patients explore feelings about their situation, including fear and helplessness. Identification of personal strengths and resources may help patients cope with the current health problems and actively participate in their care. During the identification phase, the patient, Sue, expressed fear about pain during the breast biopsy. The nurse said, "Sue, you are concerned about pain during the breast biopsy. I will talk with the surgeon about keeping you comfortable during the procedure. I will also be with you during the biopsy in case you have any questions or you begin to feel discomfort."

Exploitation Phase

During the **exploitation phase**, the nurse assists the patient to use health services. The active work of the relationship happens during exploitation. Interventions appropriate to the mutually-planned goals are carried out with ongoing assessment and re-evaluation. Sometimes, even well-planned interventions need to be reviewed, and new, more realistic goals need to be established. The therapeutic relationship allows the nurse and patient to work together during the exploitation phase. The patient uses identified strengths and resources to regain control and develop solutions.

Termination Phase

Endings are a time for review and growth. With emphasis put on the interventions of health care, the **termination phase** is often overlooked. It can be a valuable time for the patient and the nurse to examine the achievement of their goals and review their time together. The nurse uses summarization skills to evaluate the progress of the interventions toward the intended goals. This review can bring a sense of accomplishment to both parties.

Emotions are part of the ending of relationships. Caring attitudes and shared experiences can result in sadness and ambivalence at the end of a nurse-patient relationship. Termination of a relationship can awaken feelings of loss from previous relationships. Acknowledgment of these feelings is helpful in dissipating sadness and learning healthy skills for dealing with endings. The termination phase is also the time when unmet goals are identified that may require referral for follow-up care.

Resolution Phase

Ending a therapeutic relationship is always met with ambivalence. Trusting and caring relationships are some of the most satisfying parts of a nurse's job. Often, very meaningful sharing has taken place during a patient's challenging journey through illness toward health. The relationship is established with a purpose and, frequently, a time frame. For example, the nurse at an outpatient surgical center has a short time frame for the relationship with the patient undergoing arthroscopy. On the other hand, the oncology nurse has a long-term relationship with the patient with recurrent colon cancer that might end with the patient dying. Each relationship, both the short- and the long-term, requires preparation for the end or resolution.

Patients and nurses respond in a variety of ways to ending relationships. Each brings his or her prior experiences of endings and losses. When the end is nearing, patients might regress, become anxious, act more superficially with the nurse, or become more dependent. The nurse might detach and also spend less time with the patient in preparation for termination of the relationship. Any and all of these responses are normal and need to be expressed.

As the end becomes inevitable, the nurse and the patient might even become angry. The nurse becomes angry at the circumstances that will end the relationship, and the patient becomes angry with the nurse making the relationship end. Both need to express their feelings, especially reminiscing about the accomplishment of goals, the sharing of moments, and the sadness at ending the relationship. All these feelings are normal responses to the ending of a relationship, even a professional one. Nurses should not avoid the discomfort they expect to feel during these discussions, because the ending is well worth the time. The therapeutic relationship will finish with a completeness and satisfaction that is rewarding to both the nurse and the patient.

SETTING BOUNDARIES

When establishing a nurse-patient relationship, certain social parameters are set by the purpose and goals of the relationship. The therapeutic relationship is a professional relationship revolving around the patient's needs. Objectivity is important when assessing a patient's needs and providing competent and professional care. Being a compassionate nurse means being a feeling person but not being so emotionally close to the patient that objectivity is impaired.

Self-awareness allows the nurse to balance the use of the professional and personal self. For example, the nurse in an outpatient internal medicine practice has been following an elderly woman for 5 years. The nurse has cared for the patient during many stressful episodes of angina and during the loss of her husband. This patient even reminds the nurse of his grandmother. One day, the nurse observes the patient being given advice by another nurse with which he does not agree. Rather than wait for a private moment to discuss the issue with his coworker, he interrupts the conversation, corrects the other nurse in front of the patient, and gives the patient what he feels is better advice. This episode breaches at least two tenets of good communication. First, the nurse should not correct a coworker in front of a patient. This is disrespectful to the coworker. Second, the patient needs to trust her team of providers, and this encounter may make the patient feel that other people in the office are incompetent. Perhaps the nurse felt possessive or concerned about the patient's care beyond the level of professionalism and objectivity. Caring for patients can often blur the boundaries between professional behavior and emotional responses. As you grow as a person and a nurse, you will be better able to differentiate between compassionate care and over involvement with a patient that endangers your ability to provide competent, professional, and objective care.

EXERCISE

Establishing the Relationship

Break into groups of three, with one person assuming the role of the "patient," one the "nurse," and one the "observer."

- "Nurse"—Establish the relationship.
- "Patient"—Assume the role in the scenario.
- "Observer"—Give feedback on the establishment of the nurse-patient relationship and the verbal and nonverbal communication.

Take turns playing each role with the three following scenarios.

1. The patient is a 20-year-old single mother bringing her 2-month-old baby in for a series of immunizations. The nurse works full-time in the pediatricians' office, but not always with the same pediatrician.

2. The patient is a 38-year-old male arriving in the ambulatory surgical center for an arthroscopy. The nurse will be with the patient pre- and postoperatively.

3. The patient is a 28-year-old grava 1 para 0 arriving in the maternity ward in early labor. The nurse will be with the patient this shift and tomorrow on the evening shift.

Chapter 6

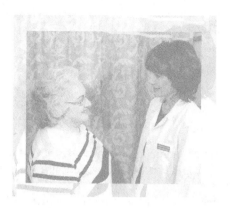

INTERVIEWING SKILLS
A Clinical Art and Science

CASE STUDY

Mrs. R. is a 57-year-old Hispanic woman who arrives in the emergency room one evening with her adult children. Her husband of 36 years passed way 2 months ago. Her children say that she has been very weepy since her husband's death. She has been holding her chest since this morning. She says that her heart aches since her husband died, and she does not want to eat. The emergency room nurse must now assess the patient's symptoms.

Nurse: "Hello, Mrs. R. I am Laurie Gardner, and I am the nurse who will be taking care of you. How are you feeling tonight?

Mrs. R.: "I am so sad without my husband." (Weeping and holding a tissue to her chest.)

Nurse: "I am sorry for your loss. You are holding your chest. Do you have pain in your chest?"

Mrs. R.: "My heart aches but it feels better when I stop and sit still."

Nurse: "Does anything else hurt?"

Mrs. R.: "My neck aches sometimes, and I feel sick to my stomach."

Nurse: "How long have you had the pain in your chest, ache in your neck, and stomach problems?"

Mrs. R.: "Since my husband died, but I feel worse since I raked the lawn this morning."

INTRODUCTION

How does the nurse begin to sift through the patients' symptoms and responses? Not only do patients present with health issues but also with their own interpretations of their health status. They come with cultural beliefs, which affect their perception of their health or illness. Although the science of nursing directs the patient interview, it is the art of nursing that derives the meaning from the patient's words. Interviewing skills are essential to understanding the patient's health and experience.

As discussed in Chapter 5, a therapeutic relationship is based on trust, empathy, and respect. The establishment of trust is particularly important when obtaining personal information from the patient as he or she will be comfortable sharing their feelings and symptoms with the nurse. Empathy allows the nurse to try to "understand exactly" the experience of the patient. Respect allows for a nonjudgmental view of the patient and his/her attitudes, values, and feelings. This chapter reviews interviewing skills that produce accurate, reliable, and complete information.

SETTING GOALS

Every encounter between a patient and a nurse begins with the establishment of the roles each party will play in the relationship. As discussed previously, the nurse has standards of care set by the nursing organizations, state laws, and the institution where he or she is employed (see Chapter 3). The patient brings expectations about the nurse's role based on public information, social anecdotes, and personal experiences. The patient may also have his or her own agenda, problems that he or she believes can be attended to by the nurse and other health care providers. Establishing the guidelines of the relationship will make the encounter more predictable and less stressful for the patient.

Within the context of establishing roles, students need to accurately identify themselves and their role to the patient, even if this feels difficult. Many patients feel that they are helping a student learn and actually enjoy the added attention provided by a student nurse. All nurses, including students, need to answer questions sensitively and honestly but admit when they are lacking answers and offer to find information from other sources. What is important is to project confidence so that the patient feels more comfortable with the nurse's abilities. Students often ask how they can display confidence when they are still learning. Remember, it is possible to be confident both in one's skills and in the ability to find information for a patient. Experienced nurses are still always learning, even after many years of practice.

The nurse also has expectations of the patient and the patient's participation in the pursuit of health. In the inpatient setting, a person walks in the door and removes his or her clothing, dons the patient uniform (the Johnny), puts his or her worldly possessions in a bag, and leaves his or her family behind. The person becomes "a patient," often with feelings of powerlessness and dependency. And yet, as health care providers, nurses expect honest answers, cooperation, and active participation from their patients. Not all patients can fulfill these expectations or even understand what is expected from them. It is important for the nurse to understand how the patient is feeling, to explain the plan of care, and to work with each patient to reach realistic and achievable goals. Nursing interventions and expected outcomes are determined by appropriate goals. Additionally, mutual goal setting helps patients feel more in control of their health and more satisfied with their care.

How to Set Goals

- Define your role to the patient.
- Establish the patient's needs and priorities.
- Negotiate and set realistic, measurable, and achievable goals.
- Ensure patient understanding.

ACTIVE LISTENING

Active listening is an interactive process between the nurse and the patient. It involves the nurse listening to the patient and actually hearing the patient's message, understanding the meaning of the words, and providing feedback about what was heard. When the patient honestly shares his or her experience, then the nurse can better grasp the current health issues, changes in functioning, and the patient's responses to the situation. More accurate information is helpful in identifying specific goals for treatment.

Body Posture During Active Listening

- Sit upright with torso facing patient, leaning slightly toward patient.
- Keep arms and legs relaxed, not crossed.
- Try to sit at eye level, maintaining direct eye contact but not staring. (Note: Direct eye contact is not always culturally appropriate and might require modification.)

- Nod or smile to acknowledge the patient.
- Relax and listen.

An important skill for nurses, active listening can be learned with practice. While it sounds simple, it requires the active suspension of the nurse's other thoughts and feelings. The focus shifts to the content and emotional content of the patient's message. Rather than judging or quickly responding with rote phrases, the nurse must listen carefully to what the patients are saying, or perhaps *not* saying, about their experience.

BARRIERS TO ACTIVE LISTENING

Many factors can influence the ability of the nurse and patient to communicate. Some are recognizable and readily changed, and others might delay communication until a more conducive situation arises. The setting, timing, and anxiety levels of the patient or the nurse can impede communication.

The **setting** should be private, so that the patient feels comfortable divulging private information. When in doubt, the nurse should ask the patient, "Do you feel comfortable talking here?" or "Where do you want to meet so we can talk?" A private setting also allows for the sharing and protection of confidential information.

Timing is very important to therapeutic communication. If the patient is not ready or able to talk, then meaningful conversation will be limited. The nurse should assess the patient's readiness to talk and the timeliness of the topic prior to initiating a dialogue. For example, if a patient has just returned to the floor after a bowel resection and colostomy creation, then teaching about deep breathing would be timely, but a discussion about changing the colostomy bag should wait until later in the hospitalization.

Anxiety can cause difficulties in listening as well as talking in any person. Patients may be nervous about their diagnosis or well-being and not be able to listen. They might try to "laugh it off" or use silence or sarcasm to avoid exploration of anxiety-producing subjects. The amount of information that the patient can process decreases with increased anxiety levels. At other times, information can lower anxiety levels, such as often happens during preoperative teaching.

Anxiety can also impair the nurse's ability to perform. The nurse may be anxious about a particular new treatment or the situation might be strenuous, such as during a respiratory arrest. For example, when a patient is physically unstable, an inexperienced nurse might become anxious and not hear the patient describing other symptoms. While there might be no way to decrease tension during certain situations, it is crucial to understand that listening and judgment can be impeded. Nurses need to use each other to validate what they believe is happening and to act as a support system during stressful situations. Asking for help, expressing anxiety, and timing meaningful conversations with colleagues can lower anxiety levels.

SILENCE

While this is a book about talking, it is also necessary to write about the uses of silence. It has been said that one cannot hear when talking. Silence can be one of the most potent parts of listening. It allows the importance of a verbal message to sink in and permits adequate time for composing a thoughtful response. Silence after discussion of a point conveys the importance of the discussed topic prior to moving on to the next subject. When the patient is silent, it might indicate that a message was powerful or emotional. Allowing the silence to continue conveys respect for the patient's response and acceptance of his or her reaction. Sometimes silence is used by patients to avoid disclosure or to avoid anxiety-producing topics (Table 6-1). Silences can become too long and uncomfortable for some people, both nurses and patients. You need to avoid breaking a silence because of your discomfort. With experience, you will come to sense when a conversation needs restarting or when words of comfort may be helpful to the patient.

The Uses of Silence

- To convey a respectful presence.
- To allow active listening.
- To permit careful composition of responses.

TYPES OF RESPONSES

Gaining more information requires active listening followed by responding. Three types of responses are useful in gathering accurate data during the assessment: restatement, reflection, and clarification. In these examples, a 71-year-old woman with a history of congestive heart failure arrives in the urgent care department complaining of shortness of breath.

- **Restatement** is an initial response that involves paraphrasing what was said. Used sparingly, restatement acknowledges that the listener has heard what was said.

  Patient: "I feel like I can't catch my breath."

  Nurse: "It is hard for you to catch your breath."

- **Reflection** involves not only restating what was said but also reflecting the emotional undertones. This technique is more helpful as the conversation develops.

  Patient: "I am scared that my breathing will never get better."

Table 6-1
How to Respond to Silence

Possible Reasons for Patient Silence	Nurse Responses
To avoid discussion	Analyze the meaning of silence. Try "You seem quiet. I'd like you to share your thoughts.
To protect oneself	Provide reassurance to the anxious patient.
To avoid disclosure of private information	Reassure the patient that you will keep the information confidential. Allow more time for the patient to develop a sense of trust.
To regroup during intense or emotional conversation	Give the patient time to regroup.

   Nurse: "You are worried that we won't be able to help your breathing."
- **Clarification** utilizes simplification and summarization to make clear, concise statements about the patient's experience.
   Patient: "Every day, I try to do my usual housework, but I have to stop and rest after a few minutes. Even getting the newspaper is tiring."
   Nurse: "Your breathing makes it difficult to do your normal activities. That must be very frustrating."
   Patient: "I don't know what I am going to do. I have tried so many medicines. Is there anything that will make it better?"

Using careful responses and active listening helps the nurse to understand the problem and assists the patient to express her concerns. This patient is not only having difficulty with the activities of daily living because of her shortness of breath, she is also frightened about the future and her treatment options. The nurse's acknowledgment of the emotional content provides acknowledgment and support. Active listening involves hearing not only the facts but also the attached feelings and attitudes.

Nurses respond to patients on multiple levels. By listening carefully and watching the patient, you can demonstrate understanding in multiple ways, while gathering information. Certain responses will be helpful in eliciting more information and validating the patient's experience. Helpful ways to respond include interchangeable and additive responses. Conversely, ignoring or minimizing the patient's experience may stunt the assessment and threaten the therapeutic relationship.

Helpful Ways to Respond

- **Interchangeable response**—You understand the patient's feelings and respond by rephrasing his or her concerns at the same level of intensity.
  Patient: "I had so much pain yesterday that I couldn't move. I was so scared."
  Nurse: "Severe pain can be very frightening."
- **Additive response**—You recognize what the patient is saying and add what you think may be concerning him or her or offer reassurance.
  Patient: "I tried the pain pills but even they didn't work."
  Nurse: "You had so much pain that you are afraid that nothing will make it better. We will plan different ways to control the pain. Let's talk about what makes the pain better or worse."

Less Helpful Ways to Respond

- **Ignoring**—You either do not hear or act as though you do not understand what the patient has said.
  Patient: "Since the surgery, I have days when the pain is so bad that I cannot get up the stairs."
  Nurse: "How is your appetite?"
- **Minimizing**—You superficially acknowledge what has been said but respond with less intensity than expressed by the patient.
  Patient: "When the pain gets really bad, I just lay on the couch."
  Nurse: "The pain can't be that bad."

Different methods of responding can be used to gather information during the assessment. For example, Mr. B., who prefers to be called Pete, is a 28-year-old man who arrives for his annual checkup with multiple vague complaints.

Pete: "I just came for my checkup."
Nurse: "How have you been?"
Pete: "I don't know. I just don't feel very hungry lately. Otherwise, I'm O.K."

Nurse: "You don't have much of an appetite. I see that your weight is down 7 pounds this year. When did your appetite change?"

Pete: "It's been going on for months. I just feel nauseous a lot. It got so bad I even tried my mother's medicine."

Nurse: "You took your mother's medicine for the nausea?"

Pete: "Yes. She has been getting chemotherapy for pancreatic cancer. They gave her medicine for nausea."

Nurse: "Your mother has pancreatic cancer?"

Pete: (Weeping quietly) "She is not doing well. We live together and every day she looks smaller to me. She has no appetite. I don't know what I am going to do."

Nurse: (Placing her hand on Pete's hand.) "I am sorry. You care a lot about your mother. It must be very difficult for you."

In this situation, the nurse listened carefully to the patient and used helpful and additive responses to reach the source of the patient's problems. Rather than skipping over the patient's first response, the nurse delved deeper into the patient's experience and found that his mother's illness could be contributing to physical symptoms. Further evaluation and physical assessment would be necessary to completely understand Pete's symptoms, but the nurse wisely listened and learned more about the patient's experience.

The ability to respond in a helpful manner with a variety of responses is a matter of experience. More experience communicating with patients improves the nurse's ability to understand their feelings and symptoms. Helpful responses elicit more information because they acknowledge the patient's experience. During the assessment, the nurse should first try reflecting or paraphrasing what the patient has said with the same level of intensity. Then the patient agrees, adds to the nurse's impression, or corrects it. Each of these responses provides the nurse with a more accurate picture of the patient's experience and, what may be more important, the patient will feel "heard." To understand each patient's symptoms and his or her responses to them is to truly understand that person and the problem. When patients feel understood, then they trust their health care provider, and they are more apt to share information that will help in their care.

OBJECTIVITY

To obtain accurate information during an interview, the nurse must be objective. What is being objective? It means trying to remove your own beliefs and prejudices from the patient's words. It also means distinguishing between the patient's interpretation and the actual symptoms. While Mrs. R. (from the case at the beginning of this chapter) is deeply saddened by her husband's death, her chest pain is the first priority in the emergency room.

While there might be multiple problems in this case, if the nurse focused only on the sadness and possible depression, then she would miss the possible cardiac origin of the symptoms.

Keys to Objectivity

- Actively listen to what the patient is saying by being quiet and observing the patient, listening to his or her words, and watching for nonverbal cues. What is not said may be as important as the spoken words.
- Provide feedback to the patient about what you have heard.
- Use phrases like "Could you tell me more about..." or "I think you said... Is this correct?"
- Let the patient know that you understand what he or she has said.

RELIABILITY

Every time patients come into contact with health care providers, whether it is a nurse, a physician, or a physical therapist, they have a different experience. They tell their story and receive various responses from providers. Patients filter some the information to fit their interpretations of their health or illness. What the nurse as interviewer tries to achieve is some objective recount of each patient's symptoms that could reliably be obtained again by another provider. Reliability or reproducibility depends on multiple factors. First, a patient might change his or her story over time, depending on the reactions he or she receives from others. Second, each interviewer has different skills at obtaining information. Last, different providers might be looking for different information: the physician might be looking for diagnostic cues (substernal pain on exertion) while the physical therapist might be gathering data about physical functioning (back strain when raking).

What enhances the reliability of information received from patients? A standardized nursing assessment form is a great place to begin as a student or new nurse. It provides questions that you can use consistently and later customize for your patients. With time, you will detect nuances in the way a patient responds: a pause that might mean the patient is unsure of how to respond or a gesture like covering the mouth meaning, perhaps, that the patient is holding back a comment.

Listening also includes looking for nonverbal cues (see Chapter 7). A nurse will also use his or her intuition based on experience to probe deeper, depending on the situation. The experienced nurse will use his or her observations of verbal and nonverbal cues to phrase the next question in the assessment or to acknowledge how a patient might be feeling.

STYLES OF QUESTIONS

Interviewing the patient requires asking questions to gather information. Most assessment forms for the collection of historical data have a combination of open- and closed-ended questions. **Closed-ended questions** usually elicit short answers or "yes" or "no" responses. Data will be consistently gathered using this sort of structured question. An example of a useful closed-ended question is: "Are you allergic to any medicines?" But to obtain a more complete assessment, you may want to ask open-ended questions that allow for the patient's response to the experience. Often, information about symptoms and feelings are better obtained with **open-ended questions**. For example, "How would you describe the pain you have been having?" instead of "Do you have any pain?" and "What other surgeries have you had?" instead of "Have you had any other surgeries?"

At the beginning of an interview it is useful to start with open-ended questions pertaining to the patient's general status and then move to the specific issues. The "w/h" questions (who, what, when, where, why, and how) are open-ended and address specific symptoms. Next, directed or closed-ended questions can provide greater detail about the specific problem. Closed-ended questions are useful in gathering factual information and summarizing what has been said.Use of "menu" questions might help the patient more accurately describe symptoms.

- General open-ended question:
  Nurse: "What brought you into the emergency room today?"
  Patient: "I have been feeling dizzy all day. I couldn't get up."
- Specific open-ended question/statement:
  Nurse: "Tell me more about the dizziness."
  Patient: "I woke up this morning and I couldn't get out of bed. I was so dizzy and then I felt sick to my stomach."
- Closed-ended directed question:
  Nurse: "You have been dizzy and nauseous since you woke up today. Have you vomited?"
  Patient: "No, I didn't throw up but I sure felt like I could, so I laid down again. I have never felt like this before."

The interview can continue, combining different question styles.

Nurse: "It's a scary feeling. When you feel dizzy do you feel like you can't get your balance or like the room is spinning?" ("W/h" question with a menu.)

Patient: "It feels like the room is spinning around me."

Nurse: "As you go from lying to standing you feel like the room is spinning around you. You feel nauseous but you haven't vomited. Do I have this right?" (Directed closed-ended question to summarize the patient's symptoms.)

Patient: "Yes, that's it."

When questioning a patient, you will develop a sense of the patient's ability to convey information. Some patients are shy and need more directed questions to help them respond. Others will ramble or be vague, and then the "w/h" questions will help target the assessment to specific issues (see Chapter 9). With experience, you will develop a sense of different communication styles and learn which questions will provide the most detailed and accurate information.

How to Proceed with an Interview

- Start with general open-ended questions.
- Move to specific open-ended questions.
- Use "w/h" questions (who, what, when, where, why, how).
- Offer a "menu" question to help direct the patient.
- Use closed-ended questions to validate the patient's description and then summarize.

TIME

The pace of modern health care does not often allow for long discussions with patients. Questions tend to be more closed-ended, or lists are used to shorten the time needed to acquire information. Many patients, like the elderly, might not be able to understand questions that convey information rapidly. If possible, time should be allotted for careful interviewing. The more accurate the assessment or interview, the easier it is to develop appropriate interventions.

SELF-REVELATION AND HANDLING PERSONAL QUESTIONS

The process of interviewing and learning about your patient is often a personal experience. Patients often share intimate details about their lives, bodies, and feelings. Sometimes they will want to understand their nurse better or ask about personal information. Sometimes they might ask questions that are inappropriate or that are too intimate to share in the professional relationship. Remember, the focus of the nurse-patient relationship is always the patient. Long-term relationships, as in a rehabilitation hospital or an outpatient oncology center, might result in some sharing of personal information by the nurse. For example, a patient with metastatic breast cancer comes to the oncology center for weekly Herceptin infusions. Over the course of 2 years, a relationship with the oncology nurse develops and sharing of some information occurs during the infusions. While these might be some satisfying moments in a nurse's career, it is important to remember, particularly for the new nurse, that the focus of care is always the patient.

Timing of self-disclosure by the nurse should be sensitive to the circumstances and the patient's personality. Sharing of personal information should occur after the therapeutic relationship is established when both patient and nurse know each other and the goals of the relationship.. In a walk-in medical clinic for urgent care, a patient asks the nurse if she has ever had abdominal pain like what the patient is experiencing. The nurse would appropriately redirect the patient saying "The focus of this assessment is to help you. Tell me more about your pain." On the other hand, if a patient with diabetes who has been in your care for 3 years arrives for a routine check-up in December and asks about your plans for the holidays, then sharing information might be appropriate. Each situation should be approached individually and sensitively in order for the patient to feel trust in the nurse's professional role.

With experience as a professional nurse, you will develop a sense of what is appropriately discussed during short- and long-term patient relationships. Self-disclosure is a gradual process that occurs in steps over time. There is often a desire on the part of the patient to know his or her health care provider. When patients ask questions about you, they often want to know the person to whom they are disclosing their private information. Disclosure and trust are closely related. When patients trust you, they will more readily and honestly talk about their issues. Sharing of more personal details, such as ages of children or favorite foods, might be appropriate in established relationships. Asking a patient for a recipe might be appropriate, but asking for advice on personal issues is not appropriate. That advice would be focused on the nurse's needs and not the patient's.

Some of the most satisfying moments in nursing care occur during long-term relationships with patients. The sharing of our mutual experiences as human beings is meaningful, but the ability to differentiate between appropriate sharing and inappropriate personal questions will grow with experience. If you are not sure about how to answer a patient's questions, then ask an experienced nurse for advice about the situation. Never share personal information with a patient if you are uncomfortable. Setting boundaries with patients will help you to develop your role and focus care on the patient.

Rules on Sharing Personal Information

- Never answer a question you feel uncomfortable about discussing in the nurse-patient relationship. Refocus the interview to the patient's needs.
- Never ask a patient for advice on personal issues.
- Never share information about another patient.

SUMMARY

Interviewing skills are part science and part art. When you are a new nurse trying to evaluate a patient's status, the possibilities seem endless. With experience, you will develop a focused approach to obtaining reliable and useful information from your patients. Using a variety of questions and responses, you will be able to streamline conversations so that you efficiently and sensitively obtain the important facts. Acknowledging the emotional undertones will help the patient feel understood and enhance the development of a therapeutic relationship.

CASE STUDY RESOLUTION

Mrs. R.'s symptoms—nausea, chest pain, and weeping—could be due to any number of problems from depression to myocardial infarction. She had actually experienced a myocardial infarction. The nurse's further questioning allowed for a more accurate description of the symptoms. Mrs. R. had an uneventful recovery from her myocardial infarction and she was referred to social services for counseling.

EXERCISE 1

Read the following interview between a nurse and a patient. Label each statement by the nurse as to the type of response or question used: closed-ended question, open-ended question, menu, interchangeable response, additive response, ignoring, or minimizing. Some statements or questions can sometimes fit into more than one category.

1. **Patient:** "I can't quit smoking!"
   Nurse: "Of course you can."
2. **Patient:** "No, you don't understand. I have tried everything, but when I am around my family smoking, I just can't help myself."
   Nurse: "It's hard to quit when your family smokes."
3. **Patient:** "I just keep trying new things but nothing works."
   Nurse: "You sound frustrated."
4. **Patient:** "I am."
   Nurse: "What methods have you tried to quit smoking?"
5. **Patient:** "I tried the patch and gum and even went cold turkey."
   Nurse: "Did the patch work for you?"
6. **Patient:** "No."
   Nurse: "Would you like to join our smoke-enders group or try the gum again?"
7. **Patient:** "I guess I need both to quit. Do you think it will work?"
   Nurse: "Let's check your blood pressure."

Answers

1. Minimizing
2. Interchangeable response
3. Additive response
4. Open-ended question
5. Closed-ended question
6. Menu
7. Ignoring

EXERCISE 2

Active Listening

Active listening is a skill that can be developed. Break into groups of two. One person be the "storyteller" and the other be the "listener." The "storyteller" shares a significant life experience with the "listener" in 5 minutes or less. Then the "listener" summarizes the "storyteller's" life experience. The "storyteller" then either validates the story or clarifies it.

- Did the "listener" accurately relay the facts of the story? What information was missing or heard incorrectly?
- Did the "listener" use attentive body language? (e.g., were his or her arms crossed? Did he or she maintain good eye contact?)
- Did the "listener" remember the feelings or emotions that were part of the story?
- Why was this experience significant to the "storyteller?"

Chapter 7

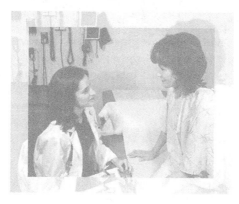

READING NONVERBAL CUES AND BODY LANGUAGE

CASE STUDY

Mr. O. is a 60-year-old man with a long history of schizophrenia who has arrived at the community health center with a cold. The triage nurse has known Mr. O. for 3 years and finds it difficult to communicate with him. Mr. O. can have unexpected angry outbursts or stare at the floor and not respond. When told that Mr. O. is in exam room 3, the nurse reluctantly approaches the room and stands in the door. The nurse crosses his arms around the chart and says to Mr. O: "How can I help you today?"

INTRODUCTION

Nonverbal communication is the process of communicating without words. It is not only the words that are used to communicate to convey meaning. A wealth of information is provided by attention to nonverbal cues, such as body language, and verbal qualities, like tone and volume. In this chapter, types of nonverbal communication meanings will be reviewed.

Body Language

People use their bodies to convey many words. Posture, the position of the arms, a gesture, or a smile can all convey a message without words. Patients might adapt certain postures that indicate vulnerability or openness to conversation. Nurses, too, might indicate their openness or interest through their posture. In the profession of nursing, body language plays an important role in building rapport with patients. Body language includes:

- Facial expressions and eye contact
- Hand and arm gestures
- Posture
- Body space
- Touch

Facial Expressions and Eye Contact

The face can convey surprise, interest, anger, sadness, joy, or fear. The facial expression can confirm the verbal message or modify it. When the facial expression and the verbal message are the same, then congruence in the words and meaning exists. The nonverbal cues reinforce the spoken words. The face can also convey strong emotions like anger and surprise, or it can be quiet or mask like. A smile usually conveys warmth and gladness when used in the appropriate circumstances. Whereas some facial expressions are easier to read, like downcast eyes and tears, others, like a blank expression, can be more ambiguous. Lack of appropriate facial expression should be noted during the nursing assessment, as some diseases like Parkinson's and some psychiatric disorders can cause a flattening of affect and minimal facial expression. Confirmation with the patient is an important component of assessing nonverbal communication because of the personal variations of expression. Statements like "You look worried to me" or "You seem uncomfortable" are ways to validate the patient's thoughts and feelings. They also denote concern and a willingness to get involved on the patient's behalf.

Cultural groups vary in their interpretation of facial expressions, especially eye contact. What may be acceptable in one culture may be offensive in another. Different cultures may interpret the raising of the eyebrows or a direct gaze as hostile or insulting. Others, like Americans, view direct eye contact as conveying interest or trustworthiness. Sometimes prolonged eye contact, especially in conjunction with physical touch, is viewed as a sign of intimacy. A downward glance might be a sign of respect, as seen in Asian-Pacific Islanders. It is important to view each patient as an individual and a product of their cultural norms when determining the appropriate methods of nonverbal communication.

Hand and Arm Gestures

Gestures with the hands and arms can tell much about the messenger. Open hands and arms may convey an openness and honesty when communicating. Folded arms and closed hands or laced fingers might indicate a reticence to talk or to divulge personal information. Crossed arms might also indicate a sense of vulnerability and a need for self-protection.

Posture

Body posture may indicate how one person feels toward another. Leaning toward another (like a nurse actively listening to a patient) demonstrates an interest in what the patient is saying. Rigid posture might convey a reluctance to engage in meaningful conversation. Crossed legs could be interpreted as crossed in self-protection, or they could be a position of comfort if all other nonverbal and verbal communication indicates openness. Tapping feet might indicate nervousness or impatience and could block useful communications. The nurse needs to be aware of the patient's body posture as well as his or her own when communicating in a therapeutic relationship.

Body Space

Body space varies with the type of relationship. Social distance is about 3 to 4 feet between people and is used in conversations between acquaintances and in business relationships. It is also used by nurses during their interactions with patients. Anxious patients might need more space to feel comfortable. Cultural differences might change the body space requirements. For example, North American, Indian, African-American, Asian, and Pakistani cultures might require greater interpersonal space than Hispanics, southern Europeans, and Arabs (Richmond, McCroskey, & Payne, 1987). Patients in pain or undergoing a procedure might need the nurse to be closer or to use touch to reassure them. Holding a hand or giving a gentle touch on the arm might make the patient more at ease during stressful times. Each patient is unique, with different body space requirements. Each situation requires assessment and adjustment to make the patient feel safe and comfortable.

The amount of body space that a person needs varies between people and cultures. Americans, Britons, and Canadians need greater personal space than Hispanic-Americans, Africans, and Arabs.

- **Intimate space** (contact to 18 inches away)—Reserved for close, personal relationships, but nurses may enter this space during care.
- **Personal space** (18 inches to 4 feet)—Used in friendships, but occurs often when delivering nursing care.
- **Social space** (4 to 12 feet)—Used in everyday life and business.
- **Public space** (greater than 12 feet)—Used during lectures and speeches.

Touch

Touch can communicate so many messages. The use of touch is the universal language of caring. It can transcend age or language differences. Reaching out physically shows concern for another human being. Touch is a powerful tool.

Nurses use touch in a variety of ways, some comforting, others as part of necessary interventions. The use of touch can reassure, calm, and support patients. For example, holding the hand of a woman in labor indicates support and caring. Nurses use touch to directly care for their patients, like during a bath or rolling them over in bed, but touch during the insertion of an intravenous catheter can be uncomfortable. A firm touch can be interpreted as controlling or hostile. The establishment of a trusting relationship prior to any invasive or painful form of touch decreases anxiety and maintains rapport.

Touch can be misconstrued as sexual by some patients. Care should be taken with these patients and the meaning of the touch should be explained to avoid misunderstandings. As a general rule, touching above the elbow, when not part of physical care, can be confusing to some patients. Careful assessment of the patients' need for space and their reaction to touch is necessary to prevent awkwardness and embarrassment.

Uses of Touch
- It can refocus patients who are rambling or self-absorbed.
- It can reduce anxiety in stressful situations.
- It can express interest in the patient's experience.
- It makes human connections and conveys caring.

CASE STUDY RESOLUTION

The nurse's words were appropriate, but everything else conveyed a reluctance to engage with Mr. O. The crossed arms and position in the doorway did not demonstrate a willingness to become involved in Mr. O.'s care. All patients, particularly those who have difficulty relating to others, need to sense attention and concern on the part of the nurse. Entering the room with an open posture would have been a better way to begin the encounter with Mr. O.

EXERCISE 1

Break into groups of three. One student be the "nurse," one be the "patient," and one be the "videographer." In 5 minutes, role play and videotape the following scenario. Have the "nurse" interview the "patient" about healthy behaviors (e.g., smoking, alcohol consumption, nutrition, sleep, checkups, etc). Then watch the videotape together, paying attention to the nonverbal behavior of the "nurse" and "patient."

- What behaviors indicate a willingness to communicate?
- What postures convey a reluctance to participate?
- What nonverbal postures did the "nurse" use?
- What nonverbal communication did the "patient" use?

EXERCISE 2

Expressing feelings without words can be a challenge. Write each of the following emotions on a separate slip of paper and distribute them. In 1 minute, act out the emotion from the paper in front of the group. You can use your face, hands, and body (like charades) but you may not make any sounds or words.

- Happiness
- Anger
- Sadness
- Frustration
- Shock
- Uncertainty
- Confidence
- Disinterest
- Reluctance
- Acceptance
- Disapproval

Questions:
- Which emotions were most difficult to portray with nonverbal cues?
- Could some nonverbal cues have more than one interpretation?
- Which emotions were easy to "read"?
- When cultural diversity might also change the meaning of nonverbal communication, how will you approach patients in your care?

Chapter *8*

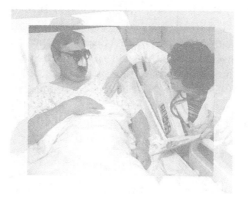

HUMOR

CASE STUDY

J.J., a 7-year-old boy, is hospitalized for a broken femur, requiring traction. J.J. rings the bell and the nurse responds to him from the intercom in the wall behind his bed. J.J. says, "What do you want, Wall?" This begins a regular joke between J.J. and the nurse. The nurse would call herself "Mrs. Wall" and J.J. found this very amusing.

INTRODUCTION

One of the most delightful aspects of human interaction is the use of humor. It can lift the spirits, free people from their everyday routines, and create human connections. Humor can put people at ease, celebrate shared victories, relieve tension, and reveal shared foibles. It is also an important communication tool in the nurse-patient relationship. When used appropriately and judiciously, humor can provide a new perspective on the challenges of life.

What amuses people is individual, but the ability to laugh is shared by all human beings.

For example, the oncology nurse in the chemotherapy suite is trying to assess Mr. R.'s bowel function, but the patient in the chair next to Mr. R. is quite close. The nurse lowers her voice to discuss stool softeners, when the adjacent patient yells out, "Oh, I used that stuff and I've been regular ever since." The two patients begin a lively discussion about different stool softeners. The humor of the situation is not lost on any of them, and a good laugh is shared by all. However, there are different types of humor and not all are appropriate in the nurse-patient relationship.

POSITIVE HUMOR

Positive humor is the kind that builds relationships and releases tension. It is constructive and joyful, creative and gentle. For example, a nurse hands a woman one johnny and tells her to leave it open in the back, and then hands her the other johnny and tells her it's the robe, so she can have an elegant, matching set. This is positive humor, based on the ridiculousness of hospital gowns. It breaks the tension of undressing and hopefully brings a smile to the patient. Nurses can use positive humor to share joy and humility. The highest form of humor is the ability to laugh at oneself. It shows perspective and reassures patients that we all have imperfections. Humor based on humility allows us to share our humaneness with others.

A patient is complaining about the hospital food, when the dietician says, "What do you want for $500 a day?"

NEGATIVE HUMOR

On the other hand, negative humor is not helpful. It makes people feel uncomfortable or defensive. It usually involves sarcasm or put-downs or includes racist or sexist undertones that might be offensive or hurtful. While it could temporarily relieve tension, it is unprofessional and disrespectful.

GALLOWS OR BLACK HUMOR

The use of "black humor" or "gallows humor" amongst the staff may provide relief during tense situations. The staff of a hospital often deals with the whole spectrum of health and illness, from spilled body excrement to nudity and death. Black humor provides a psychological escape from the harsh realities and strengthens the staff relationships. These shared experiences can provide "comic relief" from the absurd and frightening. One note: it should never be shared with the patients. For example, a joke about leaving a surgical retractor behind after a surgery is best kept within the staff.

APPROPRIATE USE OF HUMOR

When is it appropriate to use humor as an intervention in health care? Like much of life, timing is everything. It is important to understand the patient's perspective when dealing with a health problem. Try a simple joke, like the "johnny scenario," to assess the patient's response to levity within the context of the situation. Some patients and families, particularly during emergency or critical situations, will feel that their care is not taken seriously if you make a joke. Make sure the content is appropriate; that is, not racist, sexist, sarcastic, or demeaning. If you try a joke and the patient feels offended, make sure to apologize and reassure the patient that it was an attempt to be helpful or to put him or her at ease.

Often, the patient will set the tone of the conversation. He or she might joke about his or her disease by calling it a name. One female patient with chronic lymphocytic leukemia would say "Luke is back" when her white blood cell counts would start rising, indicating the need for more chemotherapy. A coworker who uses humor effectively can be an inspiration and a teacher. Try being open to different forms of interaction, including humor, to develop a style of communication with patients that is unique, effective, and rewarding.

Uses of Humor

- To begin interaction.
- To put the patient at ease.
- To convey joy.
- To lighten the atmosphere and relieve tension.
- To reveal our weaknesses and humanity.
- To acknowledge the absurdities of life.

STRATEGIES FOR USING HUMOR

- Start with gentle humor. When a patient tries to talk while you are taking a blood pressure, lift the diaphragm up like a microphone and say "What was that?"
- Try to put the patient at ease during tense situations. When the nurse has difficulty finding a good site for an intravenous catheter, she says: "Can I give you one of my veins?"
- Incorporate humor in teaching. A nurse struggling to draw a heart to explain valve surgery to a patient says, "Wait until we get to kidneys. I am good at drawing them!"

- Make a book of jokes and cartoons to share with patients. A cartoon shows an elderly woman coming in to the urgent care center. The nurse asks, "What brought you in today?" She says "I have bureau disease. My chest is in my drawers!"
- Use puppets, props, and toys, even bubbles with children (or adults!)
- Encourage a positive attitude in the patients and staff. Use group projects like decorating the department for holidays or create special days like "wear-purple-Fridays."
- Keep games like cards, electronic chess, or checkers, and funny videos to help patients pass the time enjoyably.
- Use humor with each other. The staff that laughs together is more productive, and job satisfaction and retention are higher.
- Keep jokes simple and playful with children. "What happens when ducks fly upside down? They quack up!"

Chapter 9

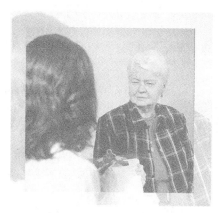

ANGER, ANXIETY, AND DIFFICULT COMMUNICATION STYLES

CASE STUDY

Debilitating osteoporosis has caused Mrs. R. to have several fractures and has limited her ability to walk. She arrives by wheelchair at the outpatient center for an intravenous infusion of pamidronate to prevent further deterioration of her bones. The nurse, who knows Mrs. R. from previous visits, arrives in the waiting room to bring Mrs. R. back for her infusion.

Nurse: "Good morning, Mrs. R. Are you ready to get started?"

Mrs. R.: "Ready? What good does this do me? You think I want to have this?"

Nurse: "You sound upset today."

Mrs. R.: "You don't know what it's like. I am just another patient to you. Get them in and get them out, right?"

INTRODUCTION

Not every patient is easy to deal with or grateful for nursing care. The stress brought on by the demands of illness can disrupt a patient's normal functioning. Personality factors, including coping patterns and attitudes, can affect how a patient responds to the challenges of life. Some patient behaviors may be challenging or even offensive to you. This chapter discusses some situations that make communication more difficult. It presents some strategies for dealing with some common patient responses to health, illness, and crises. The goal is to assess the patient's behavior and perform your nursing roles, and yet maintain respect for the patient and your own integrity.

DIFFICULT SITUATIONS

Anger

Although it does not happen often, there will be times when you will have to deal with angry patients. As in the case study, anger is often a response to fear, frustration, and/or anxiety. Regardless, it can still be uncomfortable to be the one on the receiving end of an angry outburst. Until the source of the anger is identified, you might find it difficult to deal with a patient who seems hostile.

A patient could be angry for any number of reasons. Anger might be the patient's response to loss of control or independence—common problems in hospital settings. It can be a reaction to asking the patient to disclose too much personal or revealing information. Anger might be part of how a particular personality deals with stress or loss of control. It might be a response to a similar, unresolved situation in the past. A patient might be fearful of the illness and treatment or uncertain about the future. Anger can be displaced, onto you, the nurse. Or the patient might be angered by circumstances arising out of the health care experience. Because of the variety of sources, anger must be understood as a unique response to a stressful situation and assessed individually in order to understand the behavior.

Anger is a complex emotion. Trying to understand what generated an angry response requires active listening during the outburst. This allows the emotional component of the response to dissipate. At the same time, you listen for the actual content of the message. Patients need to be heard when they are angry, and the best approach is to listen first. Then, you can reflect and restate or clarify what you heard. It is important to listen without becoming defensive, a common response. It is a natural reaction on your part to want to avoid anger or to feel personally attacked. But, you should not take the anger personally. Most of the time, the patient needs to become angry en route to coping with the situation. Occasionally, your behavior or lack of action is the source of the anger. Active listening is still the best approach to understanding the patient's point of view.

There are several ways to work through angry responses from patients. First of all, you will need to suspend your personal responses to angry outbursts. To assertively and professionally work through angry exchanges, you should begin by taking a deep breath, relaxing, and listening to the content of the patient's message. Common responses from nurses to patients' anger include disliking the patient or feeling angry or defensive when dealing with the patient. You should try to acknowledge that these responses might result from your own previous life experiences with anger. But you have a responsibility to acknowledge the patient's response and try to understand the source of the anger.

Once the problem is understood, you can begin resolving the situation. The first step is to ask the patient for clarification. For example, a patient rings the call bell and yells at the nurse manager, saying he has been waiting for at least an hour for his pain medicine. The nurse could say "I think I hear you saying that you have been waiting too long for your pain medicine. Is that right?" Next, acknowledgment of the emotional component of the message is often helpful (e.g., "You are already uncomfortable and this situation is frustrating."). Finally, you can devise appropriate solutions to resolve the issues that created the patient's response. The use of "I" statements lets the patient know that you understand the situation. Offering to work together to solve the problem could provide support and control to the patient. ("I want to make sure that you receive your pain medicine within 15 minutes of your request. Let us try...").

Dealing with an Angry Patient

- Listen actively during the outburst, letting the patient set the pace. Avoid becoming defensive, passive, or aggressive during the outburst.
- Keep the tone of your voice low and controlled.
- Avoid excessive smiling or rote responses.
- Reflect or restate what has been said, seeking clarification but explaining the reality of the situation.
- Wait for the emotional energy to dissipate.
- Offer clear, assertive ("I") responses and offer to work collaboratively to solve the problem.
- Get help or have another person present if the patient is unable to control his or her anger or if there is a threat of physical harm.

Anxiety

When patients are faced with threats to their health and well-being, a natural reaction is to become anxious. The feeling of anxiety might result from fear, frustration, conflict, or as a common response to stress. Anxiety is an uncomfortable feeling of dread or apprehension, and the source of the feeling is often unknown. Anxiety can occur on several levels. As the level of anxiety increases, the patient's level of awareness and interaction with the environment decreases.

- **Mild** anxiety is common in daily life and can be productive, even helpful, in meeting life's challenges. For example, mild anxiety can actually improve performance on an exam.

- **Moderate** anxiety can result in a decreased level of awareness and a diminished ability to pay attention. For example, the patient might not remember preoperative teaching before a major surgery if he or she is experiencing moderate anxiety. It may be helpful to the patient to have another person, like a family member, accompany him or her and to provide written information about the surgical experience.

- **Severe** anxiety produces a significantly decreased ability to focus, and interact with the environment except on a few details. Increased anxiety levels can produce physical symptoms, such as heart palpitations, sweating, dry mouth, bowel disturbances, and sleep disturbances. If the anxiety further intensifies, panic can develop, with severe incapacitation and inability to function.

Nurses are often called upon to identify and reduce anxiety. Signs and symptoms of anxiety include restlessness, tremors, hand-wringing, forgetfulness, difficulty sleeping, rapid breathing, and heart palpitations. Excessive use of the call bell and repetitive questions are examples of patient behaviors that could signify higher levels of anxiety. Identification of the source of anxiety can lead to appropriate teaching and support.

Nurses are not immune to anxiety, and many situations in health care are very stressful. Anxiety is also a very contagious emotion. It will help if you understand what triggers your anxiety. For example, some nurses find performing painful procedures, like changing burn dressings, very stressful. If this is the case, you might find talking with peers and alternating patient responsibilities to be most beneficial to you and your patients. When you separate your responses from the patients' reactions, you can intervene more therapeutically with patients and preserve your own psychological well-being.

Some of the best approaches to reducing patient anxiety are already part of the nursing role. For example, nurses are very adept at interpreting different health problems, teaching wellness behaviors, answering questions, explaining medications and side effects, and negotiating the health care system for their patients. Often, information specific to the concerns helps diffuse anxiety about the unknown. Nurses are able to be supportive and compassionate during stressful events or during the decision-making process. They can help identify what the patient perceives as threatening, assess the patient's support system and previous coping mechanisms, and plan interventions to alleviate anxiety. Remember that sometimes what patients need to do is talk, and active listening on your part may be all that they need to feel less anxious.

Strategies for Helping Anxious Patients

- Be alert to signs and symptoms of anxiety.
- Be understanding of the patient's feelings, showing concern and providing support.
- Avoid becoming tense or defensive if the patient starts complaining.
- Speak slowly and briefly, avoiding empty phrases like "Just pull yourself together" or "You'll feel better tomorrow."
- Help the patient verbalize his or her feelings and try to identify the source of anxiety.
- Do not assume you know what caused the patient's anxiety.
- Offer explanations or information if the patient has misconceptions about his or her situation.
- Assess the patient's support systems.
- Identify previously useful coping mechanisms.
- Tailor interventions to alleviate the source of anxiety where possible or support the patient through the situation.
- Refer patients with severe, unresolved anxiety for further evaluation.

Depression

The patient who appears depressed is always a concern to the nurse. Some depressive symptoms are short term and related to adjustment or changes in health or life situation. For example, the diabetic patient who has a limb amputated because of circulatory impairment will naturally be saddened by the loss of mobility and change in body image and lifestyle. Approaching depressive symptoms in this patient will be different from intervening with a patient with longstanding depression.

Signs and symptoms of depression include changes in appetite, difficulty sleeping, lack of interest in previous activities, decreased libido, crying, and slowed speech and movement. The patient might express feelings of sadness, hopelessness, futility, and helplessness. Depressive symptoms can occur during the normal grieving process, so-called "situational depression." For example, the loss of a loved one, major changes in life situation, or the diagnosis of a terminal illness can all cause these symptoms. But situational depression is time limited. The patient's symptoms gradually lift, and the patient resumes normal life activities.

More severe depression lasts longer and might not have any basis in a life event. Patients with severe depression have low energy levels and little interest in activities. They might have feelings of worthlessness and futility. One great concern is that these feelings might lead to suicidal ideation, a way to put an end to their suffering. Depressed patients who become increasingly withdrawn, agitated, or restless, or who talk about killing themselves, even jokingly, require immediate intervention.

Talking with Depressed Patients

- Initiate the conversation ("You seem unhappy today.").
- Show understanding and caring; accept all behaviors, including tears and anger.
- Focus on the patient's abilities, promoting a realistic and hopeful attitude.
- Discourage the patient from making any major life decisions.
- Encourage simple activities (like gardening, folding laundry) as the depression starts to lift.
- Take seriously all suicidal ideas and statements (like "ending it" or "doing myself in" or "showing them") and begin immediate intervention, referring the patient to the appropriate professional.

Crisis Situations

A crisis can occur whenever the normal balance of life is disturbed and normal coping skills are inadequate. There are two main types of crises: developmental and situational.

Developmental crises can occur during normal growth and development. From birth to death, normal milestones can present great challenges. Examples of developmental crises include weaning, starting school, marriage, and death of a loved one. As described by Erikson, developmental milestones are a series of crises that upset the normal balance and require new strategies to mature through the crisis. Successful negotiation of a developmental crisis allows maintenance of equilibrium and continued growth. Nursing interventions are focused on the patient's situation, past experiences and current circumstances. Developmental crises are frequently interwoven into other life events, requiring careful questioning and an individualized approach to moving through the crisis.

Situational crises arise out of external events over which a patient has no control. When a situation is unexpected, it can produce stress as the patient tries to adapt using his or her available resources. A crisis develops when the patient's usual coping abilities, personality, or other life circumstances make the unplanned situation overwhelming. Examples of situational crises include a work-related injury, house fire, car accident, or sudden illness.

Both types of crises result in predictable phases of behavior. Fink (1986) described the phases as shock, defensive retreat, acknowledgment (renewal stress), and adaptation and change. The shock phase starts when the patient is first faced with the event. The patient might feel that the event is unreal, then, soon after, feel bewildered. Suggestions from others are most helpful at this time. In the second phase, defensive retreat, the patient tries to reduce the sense of overwhelming stress with denial, anger, or wishful thinking. During the acknowledgment phase, the patient admits the reality of the situation and begins to mobilize resources and coping skills to adapt to the situation. If this phase is not successfully navigated, apathy, depression, or suicidal thoughts can develop. The final phase, adaptation and change, proceeds when the patient regains a sense of self in his or her changed reality. Anxiety and tension decrease during this phase, and help from outside sources is welcomed.

Interventions during the crisis situation require careful assessment and mutual goal planning. The assessment should include the event and its effect on the patient and family, support systems available to the patient, previous coping skills used by the patient during stressful situations, and the risk of suicidal or homicidal behavior. After the assessment, the goals of treatment are set with the patient. Nursing interventions are tailored to the individual patient and could include outside referral for ongoing therapy. Interventions are aimed at reducing the impact of the stressful event and helping those affected by the event learn new ways to cope with this and future crises (Parad, 1990).

Interventions for Crisis Situations

- Establish a therapeutic relationship that allows for open and effective communication.
- Allow the patient to express his or her feelings and talk about the events. This will help diminish tension.
- Assess coping behaviors that work for this patient. Review previous coping strategies and explore new ways of dealing with stressful events.
- Encourage the patient to seek and accept help from others. Significant others, religious affiliations, and community groups can provide additional support.
- Support the patient in the development of personal relationships. Relationships help to diminish stress and refocus the patient on rewarding aspects of life.

INTERVIEWING DIFFICULTIES

Often during the interview and assessment process, you may find it difficult to obtain information from the patient. Two common problems are vagueness and rambling discourse.

Vagueness

Vagueness makes ascertaining details about a patient's health challenging at best. Incomplete information makes identifying problems difficult and planning interventions nearly impossible. Adequate data collection is essential to accurately specifying problems so that appropriate treatment can be started.

Sometimes patients are vague because of a lack of understanding or mental acuity. On the other hand, patients might give vague answers when they are asked questions that are too broad or difficult to understand (see Chapter 6). When the patient responds with vague, nonspecific answers, you need to ask specific, directed questions to elicit more specific information. If the patient has difficulty understanding medical terms, then you can use more colloquial speech. For example, a patient might not understand the word "anticoagulant" but might understand "blood thinner." If the patient is anxious, he or she might not be able to focus and generate accurate and detailed answers. You should listen to the patient to assess his or her concerns and anxiety level, re-establish rapport, and then try to alleviate some anxiety prior to asking more detailed questions.

Vagueness might also result when patients feel threatened or do not want to divulge personal or sensitive information. If you sense reticence in your patient, you might want to back up and reassess whether trust has been established and restate your goals for helping the patient. Even then, there might be subjects that the patient does not want to discuss. Or the patient may feel ashamed of his or her feelings and your potential reaction to them. You should reaffirm your respect for the patient to relieve the shame associated with self-revelation. If the details are not necessary to the patient's immediate care, or the questions seem to be increasing the patient's anxiety, you might want to acknowledge the patient's right to privacy and proceed to other aspects of care.

Hints for Focusing Vague Answers

- Make sure a trusting relationship has been established.
- Assess patient's understanding, including hearing, intelligence, and anxiety level, with general, open-ended questions: "How can I help you today?" or "What concerns do you have today?"
- Use directed and detailed questions to help the patient focus. "Tell me more about the …(specific symptom or concern)."
- Assure the patient the right to privacy. Preface sensitive questions with "Some people feel uncomfortable talking about…"
- Remember that the interview is difficult, not the patient.

Rambling

Rambling conversation can be alternately boring or entertaining, depending on the circumstance. It can prolong data collection and result in unfocused and inefficient care. Some personalities are apt to be talkative, although excessive talking can also be an indication of high anxiety levels. If you keep the interview focused, you will obtain more accurate data. Later, as time permits, interesting conversations about the patient's experiences might provide more detailed information, and they can enrich the nurse-patient relationship.

Dealing with Rambling
- Help the patient focus on the topic at hand: "I'd enjoy talking about this, but let's return to..." or "I'd like to hear more about..."
- Clarify what you heard with the patient: "I think I hear you saying that..."
- Re-establish the purpose of the visit: "Today, we need to focus on..."

DIFFICULT BEHAVIORS

Demanding Behavior

When independent people are put in the position of dependency and uncertainty, they can feel threatened and become demanding of the staff. As patients, these people might relate to nurses with simple responses and repeated requests for services, perhaps because of increased anxiety levels or out of a need for control. They feel less threatened if they can maintain some control over unpredictable situations. Sometimes the repeated demands might make you feel inadequate or subservient. Normal responses to demanding patients are often defensive ones. But defensive postures by both patients and nurses will result in stilted conversations with little meaningful content. Nurses tend to start avoiding demanding patients, making patients perceive less care and even less control. This vicious cycle can lead to inadequate nursing care.

Similar to dealing with angry patients, your best response is one of neutrality and support, not taking offense or relating emotionally to demanding remarks. Instead, you can try using a flexible communication style, providing the patient with explanations about resources and time availability. Nursing interventions should be geared toward mutually established goals. Limit setting might be necessary if the patient's requests are extensive or burdensome to the staff.

Some Approaches to Demanding Patients
- Avoid a defensive response. Take a deep breath and listen.
- Talk in a moderate tone of voice.
- Do not engage in debating, but rather, be inquisitive and flexible.
- Explain the nurse's role and availability to the patient.
- Incorporate the patient's wishes as permitted by time and circumstances.
- Seek support from peers so that patient care is not compromised.
- Set limits as necessary to ensure safe and effective care for all patients on the unit.

Sexually-Overt Behavior

All human beings are sexual creatures. To deny the existence of sexuality is to limit the human experience. In Maslow's hierarchy of needs, sexuality is one of the basic needs, like food, air, and water. When patients enter the health care setting, they do not become asexual. They might wear unisex gowns and name bands, but they do not have their sexuality locked up with their valuable possessions. The experience of illness and disability can change how patients maintain their sexuality. Nurses need to be thoughtful and careful during this time.

Basic Rules for Communicating about Sexuality

- Maintain privacy in the physical space (closed doors and curtains).
- Reveal private patient information only as needed to those involved in care (see HIPAA Guidelines).
- Avoid making judgments about the patient's decisions, lifestyle, or values.
- Prevent shameful or embarrassing situations by providing for privacy, assessing patient readiness to talk, and referring the patient to other health care providers for discussions of sexual issues if you are not comfortable.
- Watch for cues that might indicate emotional scars from abuse, such as feelings of shame, aversion, or aggression.
- Do not assume that most adults know about sexual functioning.

Physically caring for patients can sometimes lead to confusion about sexually appropriate behavior. Physical touch is a normal part of providing a great deal of nursing care, but it can be misunderstood by some patients. Sexually explicit remarks, inappropriate touching, or making jokes that could be perceived as "off-color" might make you uncomfortable and reluctant to spend time with the patient. You should respond honestly and immediately to comments or touching that makes you uncomfortable. If the direct approach is ineffective, then talk with supervisors or the social work or psychiatry departments to develop strategies for limiting patient behavior.

Nurses need to be aware that their behavior might be inappropriate in the nurse-patient relationship or misconstrued by patients. Revealing clothes or talking about personal details of your romantic life might confuse patients and blur the lines of the professional relationship. It is important to remember that the focus of the nurse-patient relationship is the patient. When a nurse is unsure if a conversation or behavior is appropriate, the advice of a trusted colleague might provide feedback and different approaches.

Responding to Sexually-Overt Behavior

- Dress appropriately and monitor your behavior and conversation.
- Respond immediately and honestly to sexual talk or touch: "I prefer that you not touch me in that way" or "That kind of joke makes me uncomfortable."
- Set appropriate limits if patient behavior is repetitive: "If you talk that way again, your privileges will be taken away."
- Ask another nurse to be present during physical care or change patient assignments as needed to provide relief.
- Review the circumstances with a trusted colleague or supervisors.
- Collaborate with other health care providers such as the social worker for additional approaches and support.

CASE STUDY RESOLUTION

The nurse continued to wheel Mrs. R. back to a more private location and said, "Let's go back to a quieter spot to talk." Sitting in a chair beside Mrs. R., the nurse said, "Mrs. R., you are not just another patient. You seem upset today. I want to help you." With a sideways glance at the nurse, Mrs. R. said, "I was once young like you. I could walk and take care of myself. Now, I wake up and I check on what hurts today. I have to be so careful. Life just isn't fun anymore." The nurse paused, put her hand on Mrs. R.'s hand and asked, "What can I do to help?"

EXERCISE

Difficult Situations

Working in groups of three, pick one of the following three scenarios to act out. One person will be the "patient," one the "nurse," and one the "observer." Taking 10 minutes, act out the scenario.

1. Mrs. P. is a 68-year-old woman on the medical-surgical floor preoperatively for a thoracotomy tomorrow. Four weeks ago she was on the same floor for a lung biopsy, which proved positive for a non-small cell lung cancer. Today, she has made nasty remarks to the admitting nurse about the quality of care at the hospital, and now she has been standing in her doorway, across from the nursing station, for the last hour, staring at the nurses.

2. Mr. G. is a 44-year-old man with multiple myeloma who is in the outpatient unit for a monthly infusion. The nurse, a 28-year-old woman, enters the room, and the patient says, "My, aren't we looking sexy today. You look better every time I come here." When she starts to take his blood pressure, he pats her knee.

3. Sr. R. is a 72-year-old nun and elementary school teacher. She comes
   into the ambulatory care clinic with a cough. The triage nurse is interviewing the patient to get more details about her past medical history
   and current symptoms. Sr. R. very sweetly starts to answer the questions but quickly starts telling stories about children she has taught in
   the past.

After enacting the scenario, the observer will comment on the "nurse's"
approaches to the "patient." Answer the following questions as a group:

- What approaches diffused the situation?
- What comments were not helpful to the patient?
- Are there alternate approaches that would have been more useful in
  this situation?
- How does the nurse not react personally to some of the more chal-
  lenging patients?
- What resources are available to help the nurse deal with this situation?

Chapter *10*

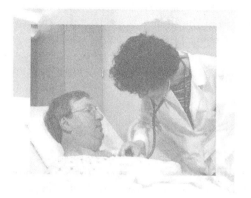

LIFE-THREATENING ILLNESS AND DEATH

CASE STUDY

Mr. T., who likes to be known as Mike, is a 57-year-old man with multiple myeloma. For the past 7 years, he has tried every possible treatment, from steroids and thalidomide to a bone marrow transplant, to manage his disease. Now, he arrives with his wife in the outpatient unit with shortness of breath, confusion, and a blood pressure of 58/38. Mike is still talking and is very clear that he does not want to be resuscitated. His wife knows that he is nearing the end of his life. She asks, "What can I expect? I just want him to be comfortable."

INTRODUCTION

For the patient and his family, the diagnosis of a life-threatening illness is a frightening prospect. A future together of shared events and family milestones is now clouded by the shadow of loss and change. Nursing interventions can have an enormous impact on the patient's adjustment to a changed future.

Nurses work in all aspects of health care in which life-altering diagnoses are given to patients, from the floor nurse who takes care of the patient before cardiac bypass surgery to the hospice nurse who helps the patient with terminal cancer reach his or her end-of-life goals. Nurses can make the process of coping and loss a more bearable and even enriching time for patients and their families.

LIFE-THREATENING ILLNESS

In a culture that fears death, the specter of dying can be overwhelming to the patient with a life-shortening diagnosis. The patient may feel emotional and spiritual distress related to the potential changes in his or her functioning and life expectancy. The disease process and treatments can affect the physical, psychosocial, spiritual, and financial aspects of a patient's life. They can experience anticipatory grieving regarding future losses and unfinished life business. You can help patients with the process of coping with illness and treatment, finding support in their loved ones, and discovering meaning in life and death.

In her landmark work, Elizabeth Kubler-Ross (1969) described the stages of death and dying: denial, anger, bargaining, depression, and acceptance. Today, they are also used to describe the process of grieving and even the acceptance of a diagnosis of life-threatening illness. While each patient is unique, you can use these stages as a framework for understanding the variety of emotions that patients might experience while trying to cope with a potentially shortened lifespan. These are not sequential stages, but rather a way to understand and then explain to patients what might be normal responses during a stressful time.

TALKING WITH THE PATIENT WITH LIFE-THREATENING ILLNESS

- Explain and answer questions about the disease and treatment, using other health care providers to help answer questions that are not within the realm of nursing. For example, the physician can discuss the prognosis or the results of diagnostic tests.
- Allow ample time for the patient to discuss his or her thoughts, feelings, and fears about the diagnosis and treatment and their impact on his or her life.
- Identify social supports that have been useful to the patient: family members, friends, coworkers, and clergy.
- Help the patient explore previous methods of coping that have been successful (e.g., talking with significant others, reading about the illness or searching the Internet for related sites, joining a support group, meditating).

- Enlist the patient and family when making decisions about care to enhance their sense of control over what can be a frightening situation.
- Observe the patient for signs of psychiatric disorders (anxiety, depression, suicidal ideas) that require further assessment, intervention, or referral.
- Provide positive feedback for the patient's use of coping strategies that work.
- Address the patient's concerns about symptom control: pain relief and control of nausea, with possible interventions if problems arise.
- Suggest support groups that are available (e.g., a breast cancer support group) to provide ongoing support from others who have experienced similar challenges.

ADVANCE DIRECTIVES

An important part of communication between patients with life-threatening illness and health care providers is advance directives. This is an umbrella term for several documents that explain the patient's wishes for cardiopulmonary resuscitation, tube feedings, and advanced life support. The documents include a living will, a durable power of attorney, and an advance medical directive. The acceptance of each of these documents varies by state. If the patient becomes unable to participate in decisions about his or her care, these documents provide the legal guidelines for health care interventions. Discussion about advance directives should occur when the patient is healthy, and not during an acute crisis when anxiety, medications, or pain can cloud decision making. Based on the patient's values, advance directives are an important means of relaying the patient's end-of-life goals when he or she is no longer able or competent to make his or her wishes known.

GRIEVING AND LOSS

The loss of a loved one can be an overwhelming event for the patient's family and friends. For example, a 56-year-old woman dies in the emergency room after a cardiac arrest. The family is in the waiting room. After the emergency room physician tells the family about the death of their loved one, the nurse is in a unique position to listen and console the family during the initial shock and grieving.

The nurse's education in communication and grieving is useful when intervening with those experiencing loss. The nurse's roles include counselor, teacher, and advocate. Experienced nurses bring skills such as identifying coping skills and supports and helping family members manage resources during times of crisis.

Family members might experience health problems during grieving that lead them to seek health care. Common physical symptoms during grieving are loss of appetite, sleeplessness, shortness of breath or tightness in the neck, a feeling of hollowness in the chest, lack of energy, dry mouth, and muscle weakness. In addition to feeling sadness, grieving people can also feel isolated, angry, guilty, lonely, numb, and/or helpless. They might cry, sigh, and feel unable to concentrate. The process of grieving has many different patterns, and unless the symptoms are overly intense or persist for a long period of time, they are normal reactions to the loss of a loved one. You help those who are grieving by listening to their feelings and memories, identifying support systems available to them, and helping them to verbalize how the loss has changed their world and expectations. Be attentive to prolonged symptoms of grieving that interfere with normal life activities like work and family roles or to suicidal ideation. Referral to other health care providers might be indicated.

The four stages of mourning have been described by Bowlby (1980):

1. Phase of numbness—General feeling of numbness and possibly denial.
2. Phase of yearning and searching—Trying to find loved one but cannot, possibly feeling or smelling them, reality starts to set in.
3. Phase of disorganization and despair—Giving up hope of finding loved one, feeling hopeless, apathetic, depressed.
4. Phase of reorganization—Seeking to remake life, establish new relationships.

Grieving is often described in stages, but the actual process is individual and unique, and may not proceed in an orderly fashion. Worden (1991) proposed four tasks of mourning. Tasks imply the "work" of grieving for the lost loved one. The work requires time, emotional effort, and concentration and cannot be hurried.

The four tasks of mourning as described by Worden are:

1. To accept the reality of the loss.
2. To work through the pain of grief.
3. To adjust to the environment in which the deceased is missing.
4. To relocate the deceased emotionally and move on with life.

COMMUNICATING WITH GRIEVING PEOPLE

- Actively listen to the person's experience, helping the survivor to express his or her feelings.
- Assess the grieving person's support systems: family, friend, clergy, or confidante with whom the person can talk freely.
- Be present and actively listen to the person's experience of grief.
- Allow ample time for the person to repeat the story of the death.

- Encourage discussion about what the future might be like without the deceased, what they will miss, what new roles the survivors will take on, etc.
- Interpret "normal" grief, allowing for individual differences: "Sometimes people hear the voice of a loved one" or "Some people miss the smell of their loved one."
- Avoid the use of rote responses like "You'll be better in no time," "It was his time," or "She's better off now."
- Suggest support groups that help family members and children who have experienced the loss of a loved one.
- Refer people with prolonged grieving, depression, or suicidal ideas to an appropriate counselor.

CASE STUDY RESOLUTION

At the nurse's request, the physician visited with Mike and his family to discuss the actual physical aspects of dying and the potential amount of time left. Afterwards, the nurse asked, "How can I help you?" Mike's wife was worried about Mike's falling in the shower. The nurse said, "Hospice services could help with daily physical care and help you, as a family, during this time." Mike's two daughters, who live nearby, visit daily and are a great source of help and support. The nurse assessed Mike's and his wife's expectations about the final days and weeks. Mike said, "I knew this time was going to come. The liquid morphine makes my breathing easier. I just like to lie in bed and watch the news anyway." Mike and his family agreed to talk with the hospice nurse that day by phone. Later that day, he slipped into a coma. Two days later, Mike died quietly with his wife by his side.

EXERCISE 1

Grief as a Personal Experience

Nurses deal with grief in their personal and professional lives. How we handle our own grief affects how we interpret the process of loss in our patients and their families.

On your own, answer the following questions and think about your answers.

- What was the first loss you experienced?
- How old were you at the time?
- How did you react to the loss?
- What was the most difficult loss you have experienced?

- Do you remember the stages of loss: numbness, yearning, disorganization, and reorganization?
- How long did it take before you felt at peace with the loss?

EXERCISE 2

Working Professionally with Grieving Patients and Families

As a group, talk about ways that nurses use their own experiences to help support patients and families during times of loss. How do nurses maintain objectivity and their own psychological well-being when dealing with grieving patients and families?

Chapter *11*

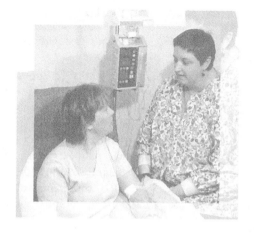

PATIENTS WITH PAIN

CASE STUDY

Bill is a 42-year-old man who is experiencing discomfort from his naso-gastric tube. It has been 48 hours since he had an exploratory laparotomy for small bowel adhesions. Bill is complaining that he feels like he cannot swallow—as if something is stretching his throat, causing him painful swallowing and coughing. The surgeon had made rounds that morning and had talked briefly with Bill about how he was feeling. Bill described the pain in his throat, but the surgeon felt that this was normal discomfort from the naso-gastric tube. After the surgeon left, Bill rang his bell to talk with the nurse about his pain. He was angry and discouraged that the surgeon had not seemed to listen to him. While nasogastric tubes can cause some discomfort, the nurse is wondering about the amount of discomfort Bill is experiencing. He goes to Bill's room to discuss the issue. When the nurse asks him to rate his pain on a scale of 0 to 10 (0=no pain, 10=worst pain of his life), Bill rates the pain on swallowing as a 7 to 8. With such a significant amount of pain, more would be expected, the nurse decides to pursue a more thorough evaluation of Bill's pain.

INTRODUCTION

Pain is whatever the experiencing individual says it is, occurring whenever he/she says it does—Margot McCaffrey, 1968

Pain is experienced by all human beings at some time in their life. It is a subjective experience of discomfort that can only be described by the one experiencing it. You cannot see or feel another person's pain. While you might have experience with other patients with similar surgeries and conditions, the patient is the sole authority on the experience of pain. You must not only accept the patient's description of the pain experience, but also convey a nonjudgmental attitude. When you accept another's experience, then the patient feels validated and understood and is more apt to share his or her feelings. Communicating with the patient in pain requires you to forget preconceptions about expected or even acceptable "pain experiences" and listen to what the patient is saying.

Pain is one of the most common reasons that patients seek health care. It can vary considerably between individuals, even if they have had the same surgery or disease. Many factors influence how a patient responds to pain. Age, cultural values, sources of support, and anxiety levels can affect the reaction to pain. To assess a patient's pain, you should use the appropriate approach, depending on the circumstances.

ACUTE PAIN

Acute pain is relatively brief in duration and diminishes as healing occurs. For example, the postoperative patient usually has acute pain and needs quick assessment and appropriate intervention. Treatment for acute pain is instituted quickly, before pain levels rise. Early intervention not only provides more comfort but also results in lower medication requirements with fewer side effects, earlier mobility, and fewer complications (Kazanowski & Lacetti, 2002).

QUICK PAIN ASSESSMENT

- **Intensity of pain**—Use a pain intensity scale, either verbally or visually, to have the patient rate his or her pain from 0 (no pain) to 10 (the most extreme pain he or she has experienced) (Figure 11-1).
- **Location of pain**—Ask the patient where he or she feels the pain, making sure it is appropriate to the surgery or trauma. If not, assess for other precipitating factors. For example, post-appendectomy pain would be expected in the lower to mid-abdominal area, whereas calf pain with flexion in the same patient would require further assessment.

0	1	2	3	4	5	6	7	8	9	10
No Pain		Mild Pain		Moderate Pain		Severe Pain		Extremely Severe Pain		

Figure 11-1. A sample pain intensity scale.

- **Quality of pain**—Help the patient use descriptive adjectives to describe his or her pain, such as burning, shooting, wrenching, crushing, aching, sharp, or piercing. Use the patient's description when documenting in the chart. For example, a patient with herpetic shingles may describe his or her pain as burning or searing.
- **Physical assessment**—Identify the objective signs of pain by visual inspection (for redness, swelling, drainage), auscultation of bowel or lung sounds, and palpation, if appropriate, for tenderness or exacerbation of pain.

Quick assessment of pain in postoperative patients or those in the emergency room allows for more rapid intervention. The key to communication with patients in acute pain is assessment, intervention, and then, frequent reassessment of the symptoms and pain relief to determine the effectiveness of the treatment and changes in their condition.

CHRONIC PAIN

For patients with **chronic pain**, a more detailed pain assessment allows for a comprehensive history of the patient's experience of pain. Chronic pain can occur because of gradual deterioration of normal tissues (like osteoarthritis), or it might linger after an acute injury (like phantom pain after an amputation). A thorough pain assessment addresses not only the intensity, location, quality, and physical cues of pain, but also previous pain-relieving methods, medications, the efficacy of previous interventions, the effect of the pain on his or her daily living, coping mechanisms, and the meaning of pain in his or her life. Chronic pain is often viewed by the patient as irreversible and meaningless. A 64-year-old woman might feel that living with the pain of arthritis is just part of growing older, whereas a younger person with persistent joint pain might feel that it interferes with his or her ability to function at home during athletic activities or at work. Remember that each patient's experience of pain is unique, and the patient is the authority on his or her pain.

The sensation of pain can be based on the underlying pathophysiology.
- **Nociceptive pain** arises directly from damaged tissues, like the pain from a burn to the skin. Nociceptive pain can be described as aching, throbbing, or gnawing.

- **Visceral pain** arises from deep tissue organs and may be poorly localized. Appendicitis is an example of a condition that can have a variety of presentations, from periumbilical pain to nausea.
- **Neuropathic pain** arises from damage to nerves and can be experienced as burning, aching, lacerating, or pricking.

Careful assessment of the patient descriptions of the type and location of pain are critical to appropriate pain management.

PAIN ASSESSMENT

- Location of pain—Have the patient not only describe but point to the area where he or she feels the pain.
- Intensity of pain (using a pain scale of 0 to 10).
- Quality of pain (using descriptive terms, as in the Quick Assessment Tool).
- Time of onset and duration and constancy of pain.
- Precipitating factors—Eating, motion, and relation to other bodily functions, like breathing, bowel movements, or coughing.
- Alleviating factors—What lessens the pain, for example, position, medications (type, frequency, effect), heat or cold, change in activity, medications, massage.
- Associated symptoms like nausea or dizziness before, during, or after pain.
- Effects of pain on daily functioning, for example, eating, working, sleeping, ambulating.
- Meaning of pain to the patient, for example, aging, worsening illness, display of weakness, fear of pain.
- Coping mechanisms the patient uses to deal with the pain.

PAIN MYTHS

Many patients avoid describing their pain because of various fears that are often unfounded. For example, one myth about pain medicines is that they are all addicting, especially narcotics. Other concerns based on fallacies include:

- Pain as a sign of weakness or a "bad" patient.
- Worries about drug tolerance.
- Fear about side effects.
- Belief that pain is to expected with a certain disease or procedure.
- Fear of injections.

The assessment of the patient's attitudes toward pain and pain relief will help in obtaining an accurate assessment, educating the patient, and customizing the interventions to achieve comfort.

PAIN MANAGEMENT

Successful pain management requires matching the interventions to the patient's pain experience. The choice of drug and dosage is tailored to the patient's needs. Frequent reassessment of pain relief from interventions and drug side effects will provide consistent control, customized dosaging, and minimization of side-effects. Communication with the patient and family about expected results, potential side effects, and follow-up will provide the necessary continuity and compliance with the pain regimen.

CASE STUDY RESOLUTION

The nurse decided to further assess Bill's pain. With a penlight and a tongue blade, he asked Bill to open his mouth. There, in the back of the oropharynx, the nasogastric tube was looped around instead of going straight down. The surgical resident was paged and told of the situation. As Bill had started to pass flatus that day, an indication of renewed bowel function, the resident gave the order to have the tube discontinued. With the nasogastric tube out, Bill felt complete relief and gratitude.

EXERCISE

Accurate assessment of pain is critical to planning appropriate interventions.
- As a group, think of some descriptive adjectives for pain, from either personal experiences or clinical ones. Write the words on the board. Describe the situation or the patient who used these words.
- Think of a personal experience where perhaps your experience of pain was not believed. How did this make you feel? What did you think about the person who did not "hear" you? How do nurses maintain an open mind about patients' descriptions of pain?

Chapter *12*

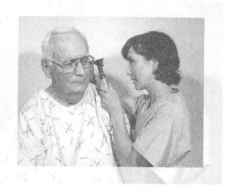

PHYSICAL IMPAIRMENTS TO COMMUNICATION

CASE STUDY

The student nurse comes out to the desk on the rehabilitation floor of a skilled nursing facility looking for the clinical instructor. She is caring for Mr. G., a 74-year-old man, who has had a stroke and can only communicate by sounds. His ability to control his emotions has also been affected by the stroke and he is frequently angry. Now, he is in the facility recovering from a below-the-knee amputation. Mr. G. is yelling loud enough at the student to be heard at the desk.

INTRODUCTION

How difficult it must be not to have the usual methods of communication! Relaying messages through words and gestures is normally wrought with mis-understandings. Imagine how complicated it would be if your ability to communicate with others was compromised. Communication deficits might last for brief periods of time, like during postoperative intubation, or become permanent changes, like hearing loss or blindness. It is important to remember is that each patient will try to adapt to the deficit. The nurse's role is to use the patient's abilities to communicate and maximize his or her independence.

GENERAL WAYS TO MAXIMIZE COMMUNICATION

- Learn the patient's communication techniques, for example, sign language, hearing aid, or family member who interprets the meanings of words.
- Allow ample time and pre-arrange for interpreters or family members to be present, if necessary.
- Place yourself at face level with the patient so he or she can see your mouth and facial expressions.
- Speak distinctly and slowly, using a moderate tone.
- Provide paper and pencil or word boards to help the patient communicate, and provide written material to the patient as appropriate.

COMMON DEFICITS

Speech and Language Deficits

Speech and language deficits can occur as part of the developmental process or as a result of illness. Deficits can occur in the receiving and the expressing of information. Language is our basic way of communicating with the world: both receiving information and conveying to others our needs and feelings.

Aphasia

Aphasia is a neurological condition in which the language function is defective or absent. There are three general types of aphasia:
1. **Expressive or motor aphasia**—Words cannot be expressed or formed.
2. **Receptive aphasia**—Language is not understood.
3. **Global aphasia**—Includes both expressive and receptive deficits.

To develop the best communication strategies for patients with aphasia, you need to understand the individual patient and his or her abilities. Assess the type of aphasia and methods used for communicating to plan the most appropriate nursing interventions.

Interventions for Communicating with Aphasic Patients
- Allow ample time for patients to formulate thought and receive information.
- Focus on those abilities that the patient has to communicate.
- Use touch, facial expressions, and sounds.
- Supply alternate methods, like written words, if current methods fail.
- Avoid prolonged conversations. Keep it short and to the point.
- Praise the patient's efforts and use humor to provide relaxation when communication becomes difficult.

Hearing Loss

Hearing loss can be a part of normal aging or the result of trauma or illness. Hearing allows the listener not only to receive verbal messages, but also to interpret sounds in the environment. Cues in the environment such as a ringing phone or a car honking might not be heard. Relationships with others are affected by hearing loss, as the person with the hearing deficit might not only miss the words, but also be unable to detect subtle changes in voice, like pitch, tone, or volume.

Assessment of hearing loss is important to planning communication. Knowing the age of onset, type of loss, and aids used will help you plan the appropriate interventions. Deafness in childhood affects speech development, making communication with others even more difficult. Children with hearing and speech deficits might use sign language to communicate. Older people might have difficulty handling hearing aids because they cannot maneuver the hearing aids or tiny batteries, and, as a result, might not wear them. Or they might not use their hearing aids because the aids amplify too many sounds.

Interventions for Communicating with Patients with Hearing Loss

- Use the method that works best for your patient: hearing aid, sign language, written words.
- Arrange for interpreters or family members to explain the patient's methods of communicating and refer to an audiologist, if necessary.
- Help patients use hearing aids, assess whether the hearing aid is working properly.
- Speak in a moderate, even tone; do not yell.
- Face the patient when talking so he or she can see your mouth and facial expressions.
- Consult with speech therapy to learn the best communication strategies for your patient.

Vision Loss

Vision loss, or blindness, causes communication deficits because vision allows people to see the speaker and his or her facial expressions and gestures. Vision loss puts the patient at a disadvantage when communicating, because the whole message is not received. The patient often feels isolated and vulnerable. Assess the patient's vision loss, including the type of loss (light, shadows, complete) and types of aids used (Braille, cane, glasses).

Interventions for Communicating with Patients with Vision Loss

- Alert the patient when you approach and state your name.
- Do not speak loudly or overly enunciate.
- Orient the patient to the surroundings, mentioning furniture, steps, or changes in terrain in advance.
- Offer your arm to the patient who is navigating new surroundings.
- Have other personnel introduce themselves to the patient when they enter the room.
- Explain procedures in advance, so the patient knows what to expect.
- Describe what you are doing when you are with the patient.
- Tell the patient when you are leaving the room.

Sensory Deprivation in Intensive Care Settings

Intensive care units, emergency rooms, and recovery rooms can be strange and frightening environments for the patient. Unfamiliar surroundings, noises, and equipment can be disorienting.

Patients may also be in pain, intubated or medicated—all of which may prevent communication. The nurse's role is the "anchor" in a bewildering setting, providing orientation and comfort to the patient, especially when immediate family might be visiting for only a few minutes.

Intensive care in a room without windows, with a great deal of extraneous sounds and personnel, can disorient the patient. Assess the patient's orientation and mental status frequently to understand what the patient needs. Tell the patient frequently the date, time, environment, and care givers, to help the patient feel less fearful.

Interventions for Communicating with Patients in Intensive Care Settings

- Introduce yourself and speak as though the patient hears everything. Stories abound about patients' memories of health experiences when they seemed unconscious.
- Orient the patient frequently to the surroundings, explaining sights and sounds, date and time, and health care staff.

- Give explanations about procedures before they occur and explain different sights and sounds that the patient might experience.
- Provide information to the patient about his or her progress.
- Even if the patient cannot speak, carry on a one-way conversation.
- Encourage the patient and/or family to display meaningful items like photographs or simple objects from home.

CASE STUDY RESOLUTION

Student: "I don't know what to do. I have tried to find out what he wants but he just keeps yelling at me. What am I doing wrong?"

Instructor: "Let's go see Mr. G., and maybe we can figure it out."

Student: (In Mr. G.'s room) "Mr. G., how can we help you?"

Mr. G. shakes his head, yells again, and points at the bed.

Student: "It seems that something is wrong with the bed or bedding. Would you help me roll him over and I'll smooth out the sheets. Mr. G., we are going to fix the sheets."

As they roll Mr. G. on his side, the student finds the remote control to the television under his sacrum. The skin around the area is indented from the remote.

Mr. G. gives a relaxed sigh and reaches over and kisses the student's hand.

EXERCISE

What is it like to lose your hearing or sight? Break into two groups.
- Group 1—Put cotton balls in your ears (hearing loss group).
- Group 2—Wear blindfolds (vision loss group).

Break into pairs. For the Group 1 ("hearing loss") student, guide your "vision loss" student around the room and down the hall without saying who you are. After one trip, sit down and describe your experiences to each other. Do not remove the cotton balls or blindfold.
- How did it feel to be unable to see the environment?
- How did the guide help the "vision loss" student negotiate the trip?
- Did touch help?

For the Group 2 ("vision loss") student, whisper a message to the "hearing loss" student.
- How long did it take for the "hearing loss" student to understand the message?
- In what other ways can messages be communicated?

Chapter *13*

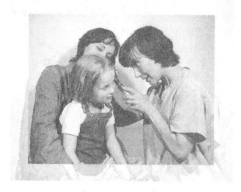

DIFFERENT AGE GROUPS

CASE STUDY

B. is a 15-year-old young man who arrives in the emergency room after a witnessed seizure at a friend's house. Disoriented and agitated, B. is not allowing the nurse to put in an intravenous line. He is physically struggling with the nurse and is quite strong. The nurse says; "B., I have to put in this I.V. and take some blood work. If you don't hold still, it will take longer and hurt more." He still refuses to let the nurse touch him.

INTRODUCTION

Talking with different age groups requires special techniques and a solid knowledge base about developmental stages. This book primarily deals with communicating with adult patients. While whole books are devoted to talking with pediatric or geriatric patients, this chapter covers the basic ways to communicate with different aged patients in health care settings.

Children need specific communication skills, depending on their stage of development. Human development has fascinated many researchers and theorists. Erikson's developmental stages were reviewed in Chapter 2. Another theorist, Jean Piaget (1972), examined the cognitive development of infants and children. Piaget saw intellectual growth as the result of interactions between the child and the environment. He perceived four stages of cognitive development.

1. **Sensorimotor stage**—The infant up to age 24 months uses the senses and motor activity to solve problems with the environment. The child gains motor control and learns about the physical environment.

2. **Preoperational stage**—Children from ages 2 to 7 years are developing verbal skills. Within the second stage, the toddler enters a substage, **preconceptual**, and begins using words as symbols. The preschool child in the next substage, **intuitive**, increasingly uses symbols, but is very concrete in his thinking. This stage is characterized by egocentrism; the child is unable to grasp another's point of view. In Erikson's scheme, the goal of this stage is to develop a sense of initiative through trying new actions and ideas.

3. **Concrete operational stage**—Piaget describes children from ages 7 to 12 years dealing with more abstract concepts like mathematics and cooperative relationships.

4. **Formal operational stage**—Young adolescents (ages 12 to 15 years) develop logical reasoning and the ability to think about the world of possibilities, and not just reality. Adolescents also develop certain behaviors like intolerance and introspection.

Communication must be age-appropriate and familiar to the child. In the health care setting, the parents are a good source of information about their child—their personality, fears, and needs. They can provide cues for younger children, like commonly used words for toileting. Parents are also the best care providers for infants and toddlers. Here are some age-appropriate strategies for communicating with different age groups.

INFANTS (BIRTH TO 12 MONTHS)

- Try to meet the infant's needs as quickly as possible.
- Use nonverbal communication: stroking, touching, holding, and motion (like rocking) to comfort and reassure the infant.
- Speak softly and smile often as infants respond best to high-pitched, gentle tones.
- Try to maintain the infant's normal routine: mealtimes and sleep schedule.
- Keep parents nearby so the infant can see them, especially for infants aged 9 to 18 months when "stranger anxiety" is present.

- Involve parents in calming the infant, as well as feeding, changing, and bathing.
- Communicate with play (peek-a-boo, rattling toys) if the infant is receptive.
- Avoid overstimulation when an infant is in physical distress or withdraws.

TODDLERS (AGES 1 TO 2)

- Use the child's name for himself or herself.
- Learn and use the child's words for toileting, eating, and bathing.
- Keep messages short and clear.
- Allow for mobility, sitting up, or walking, especially after procedures.
- Use nondirected messages to allow child control and independence, such as offering choices.
- Remember that protest behavior (like temper tantrums) can be used to deal with stress.
- Allow the child to use familiar objects, like a blanket or teddy bear, to make him or her feel safer, especially during stressful situations.
- Prepare the toddler for painful events just before they occur, and support and reassure him or her afterwards.
- Recognize regression and separation anxiety as normal toddler responses to stressful situations.

PRESCHOOLERS (AGES 3 TO 5)

- Use simple words and short phrases—preschoolers have a short attention span.
- Speak in a soft, low voice.
- Maintain some eye contact if it is tolerated by the child.
- View separation anxiety, regression, fantasy play, and projection as common responses of preschoolers to stress.
- Explain interventions using play therapy, or imagination: "The doll will feel a cold liquid on her leg."
- Provide choices, for example, "Do you want cereal or scrambled eggs for breakfast?"
- Allow children to draw what is on their mind

SCHOOL-AGE CHILDREN (AGES 6 TO 12)

- Use some of the child's vocabulary in explanations.
- Draw figures to demonstrate anatomy and procedures.
- Include the child in discussions about his or her care.
- Respect the child's privacy, there may be topics he or she won't discuss at the moment.
- Use third-person conversations to prompt communication ("Some kids don't like to...).
- Assess the child's perception of the situation prior to beginning an explanation.

ADOLESCENTS (AGES 13 TO 18)

- Take time to establish rapport by listening and remaining nonjudgmental.
- Reassure the adolescent about confidentiality within limits.
- Allow the adolescent to participate in decisions about care, using both concrete and abstract terms, encouraging the adolescent to become responsible for his or her body.
- Use correct anatomic terms about conditions and tests.
- Avoid an authoritarian style allowing the adolescent to talk.
- Respect the patient's privacy, allowing for physical privacy and modesty.
- Regard each adolescent as a unique individual despite his or her dress or appearance.
- Encourage but never force adolescents to disclose their health concerns with their families, evaluating the need for disclosure if the adolescent is in immediate danger.

ADULT PATIENTS

- Recognize that intergenerational differences might exist between the patient and the nurse; respect the patient's point of view.
- Listen to the patient's historical narrative, as time permits. It paints a picture of his or her life experiences, personality, strengths, and challenges.
- Avoid overly technical terms by assessing what the patient understands and rephrasing explanations of medical terms and interventions to the patient's level.

- Avoid using patronizing names like "Granny" and "Honey." Always start with the formal (Mr., Mrs., Miss, or Ms.) and then ask what the patient prefers to be called.
- Be aware that some adults might use a patronizing tone with younger nurses. Be respectful but knowledgeable, reaffirming your training and expertise.
- Allow extra time for teaching about tests or surgeries and medications. Go at a slower pace and reassess understanding regularly.
- Give the patient any opportunity to make decisions independently, as appropriate.

CASE STUDY RESOLUTION

This is a difficult situation, because the nurse does not want to use physical restraint, but he understands that B. is post-ictal and somewhat disoriented. When the parents arrive, the nurse explains the situation to them. The mother offers that B. has always hated needles and she asks why the I.V. is necessary. After the nurse explains the need for blood work and intravenous access, he says, "Would you come with me when I talk with B. about the need for the tests. I don't want him to feel that we are ganging up on him. We just want to help him." B., although 15 years old, is frightened and relieved to have his parents present. The nurse explains the need for the I.V. again with the parents present, confirming to B. that this is required. He agrees to the I.V. if his mother can stay with him. Luckily, the line is inserted on the first try, and B. seems calmed by his mother's presence. and touch The nurse appropriately used the parents to facilitate communication and the necessary interventions.

EXERCISE 1

Older patients frequently bring a litany of medications that they take or have used in the past. Some remedies might be folk or herbal remedies. Some might be approaches to staying healthy that do not fall in the category of medicines, like a shot of whiskey every night. What approaches can you use to provide accurate information about their current medications? How will you maintain a current list of medications for the patient? How will you know whether they are taking the medications as prescribed?

Exercise 2

While you may not have been in a pediatric clinical setting, you probably remember an instance where a child (brother, cousin, niece) needed to do something that he or she did not want to do. As a group, use the blackboard to list different approaches by age group (infant, toddler, preschooler, school-age child, and adolescent). What approaches, both serious and humorous, facilitated the necessary action? What approaches usually did not work?

Chapter *14*

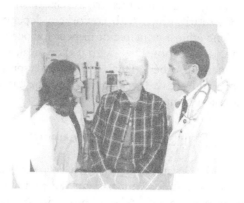

COMMUNICATING WITH PEERS AND OTHER HEALTH CARE PROVIDERS

CASE STUDY

Rose L. is the nurse manager on the rehabilitation unit of a skilled nursing facility. It has been a very busy day shift with multiple transfers and discharges, none of which went smoothly. Now, she has a pile of forms and several phone calls to complete before going into report. Tom S., a nursing assistant on the unit, comes into Rose's office and says that Mr. R. in Room 202 is complaining because his medication is an hour late, and Tom is sick of being yelled at by Mr. R. How can Rose meet the needs of the patient and the staff?

INTRODUCTION

Every working day, you communicate the needs of your patients to others: other nurses, physicians, secretaries, and therapists. As a nurse, you fill a unique role in health care as the coordinator of services for the patient. Communication with other health care providers, just like with other people, can be challenging at times. Just as each patient brings an individual set of needs, experiences, and emotions to a relationship, so does each provider. Successful relationships with coworkers depend on good communication skills. The ethical principle of respect for persons (see Chapter 3) is also relevant in relationships with other health care providers. Respect, fair treatment of others, feedback, integrity-preserving compromise, collaboration, and active listening provide the building blocks for solid professional relationships.

BUILDING RELATIONSHIPS

Whether riding in the elevator or using e-mail, you communicate with colleagues to provide good care for your patients. As in any business environment, it is better to establish solid relationships with coworkers before you need something or a problem arises. Then, you are not just a voice on the other end of the phone asking for supplies or changing an order. You are Melissa Jones, the nurse manager on the sixth floor. The best working environments encourage coworkers to know each other. All good relationships depend on good manners and communication skills.

Ways to Build Professional Relationships

- Try saying "hello" or at least smiling at everyone you meet at work.
- Introduce yourself and explain your role and job site before asking for advice, changes, or services.
- Be a supportive and encouraging coworker. Congratulate coworkers on accomplishments, give positive feedback for a job well done, offer assistance whenever you can.
- Work to build rapport in your department and workplace. Attend rounds, have coffee with different coworkers, provide an in-service on your floor.
- Use common sense in your dealings with colleagues. Praise them in public and criticize them in private.

NURSING ROLES

Defining the nurse's roles within the health care system is necessary to define the independent and collaborative nature of nursing care. Some overlap of responsibilities occurs between nursing and other health care professions. While collaboration is an important part of all jobs in health care, nurses have some special roles when communicating on behalf of their patients. These include:

- Patient advocacy
- Coordination of care
- Delegation and supervision

- Consultation
- Collaborating with peers

Patient Advocacy

Nurses have a history of advocating for the needs and interests of their patients. The word **advocacy** comes from Latin roots meaning "to summon a voice." To advocate means to defend one's own interests or to plead on behalf of another's cause, but nurses actually have a dual role in terms of patient advocacy. They work on behalf of their patients' interests and they also teach patients how to advocate for themselves.

Navigating the health care system can be complicated and frustrating. Patients often require assistance making informed decisions about their health care. Nurses are in the position to help patients find information about their health, make informed decisions, deal with employers, and negotiate with reimbursement agencies. The nurse's role requires an understanding of the communication and negotiation skills that patients need to navigate in the complex system of health care services and reimbursement.

Maintaining the rights of the patient has long been part of the nursing role. Nurses give "voice" to the patient's needs and concerns. Earlier in the book, patients' bills of rights were discussed (see Chapter 3) as one means to communicate the patients' rights within an institution, with an insurance company, or in a particular state. Nurses help patients negotiate the system in many ways, like providing health care information and interpreting medical terms. You, as a nurse, can also teach patients how to "self-advocate" within the health care system and with insurers. It is very empowering to patients and their families to know how to obtain information relevant to their health and treatment, how to negotiate with providers and insurers, and how to make decisions that are personally, culturally, and medically appropriate.

Coordination of Care

Caring for a patient often requires multiple health care agencies working together. Coordination of care between two or more agencies requires ongoing communication. During the patient assessment, you might identify health care needs that extend beyond the scope of your care. For example, an elderly woman is being discharged to home from the skilled nursing facility, after rehabilitation following hip replacement surgery. The nurse realizes that the patient lives alone and makes a referral to the visiting nurse to provide a home health assistant to help her with self-care. At other times, referrals are made by the physician for other services outside of the agency or institution. Collaborative discharge planning alerts the nurse or social worker to the need for additional outpatient services. Nurses can coordinate care between health care agencies by asking the right questions of the agency on behalf of the patient.

- What services are provided by the other provider or agency?
- What are the financial arrangements, and are they compatible with the patient's resources?
- How does the patient communicate with the agency?
- How will the patient get to the agency?

Delegation and Supervision

Collaborating with other health care providers often includes delegating care to other personnel. Nursing assistants and unlicensed assistant personnel provide delegated nursing tasks so that the professional nurse has more time for other activities. Delegation is the transfer of responsibility for the performance of a task to another person. You should know the capabilities of other personnel prior to delegating an activity. Likewise, you need to establish a method for communicating (written or verbal) the completion of the task and other relevant information.

For example, a nurse is supervising the evening shift in an assisted care facility and needs to delegate evening care and medication administration so she can deal with a sick resident. The supervising nurse must know the Nurse Practice Act in her state and the appropriate roles of the other personnel. She is responsible for assessing the knowledge level of unlicensed personnel, educating them if required, delegating the task, overseeing the activity as necessary, and then evaluating and documenting the outcomes (Boucher, 1998). Then she can delegate appropriate activities to meet the needs of the patients on the unit.

Consultation

Nurses consult with a variety of health care providers to provide the appropriate care for their patients. Consultation optimizes interventions and outcomes and enriches professional relationships. It can include calling the physical therapist for range of motion exercises for a patient after a cerebral vascular accident or referring an outpatient with wound care needs to a visiting nurse. Dieticians can assist with intake assessments and teaching for the patient with newly diagnosed diabetes. Using the expertise of other professions is essential to providing the optimum care for the patient.

Collaborating with Peers

Peer relationships provide opportunities for support and growth in the working environment. The profession of nursing values the contributions of other professions in helping to provide the best care and outcomes for patients. Cooperation with other health care providers includes consultation, collaboration, delegation, and conflict resolution. (For more on conflict resolution, see Chapter 15.)

Collaboration within nursing is essential to meeting the needs of the patient and the community. Nurses working together on staff meetings and patient rounds share their perceptions and wisdoms to enhance team decision making and support their colleagues. Sometimes collaboration occurs informally at the bedside, as when two nurses work to move a patient. On a larger scale, patient rounds and nursing conferences help to expand the knowledge of the entire staff or profession.

While many people assume that nursing means clinical patient care, it should be remembered that nurses in education, administration, and research all play important roles in directing and enhancing nursing care. Nurse educators not only train future nurses, they are also directly involved in promoting professional care through their student and staff interactions. Nursing administrators provide the vital link between hospital administration and direct clinical care. Most have been involved in caring for patients and understand the needs of the nursing staff and the environment of patient care. Nurses involved in research help to expand the knowledge base of nursing and health care.

ASSERTIVENESS SKILLS

Assertiveness is one skill used to effectively communicate your thoughts and feelings. Sometimes, the adjective **assertive** is associated with negative behaviors like being "pushy" or "uppity." Issues of sexism, power, and personal rights can confuse both the sender and the receiver of assertive messages. To convey important points, you must have a sense of yourself and understand your audience, so that the message comes across with a combination of honesty and tact. Speaking assertively does not violate the rights or integrity of others.

Assertiveness is not to be confused with aggressiveness, in which messages can come across as angry, hostile, or offensive. Yet, it is not passiveness, in which you might undervalue your contribution or yourself and layer your message with conditions or apologies.

Assertiveness is:

- Clear and direct statements
- Respectful of the rights of others and self
- Honest and genuine
- Firm and positive
- Not apologetic
- Specific to the situation

Using assertiveness skills allows you to confidently express your thoughts and beliefs. These skills are useful both personally and professionally. Patients will find your messages clearer and more understandable. Other health care providers will respect you more as a nurse and value your contribution. Personally, you will have a better sense of yourself and convey that to the people you encounter at work and in life.

Learning to act assertively requires learning new behaviors for approaching situations. This might not be easy at first. Many students feel unsure of themselves and their clinical knowledge. That will change with time and practice. Keep the following in mind as you try to understand others' responses.

- Every person responds differently to situations. What makes one person angry may make another passive or defensive. "Strive to understand, then to be understood." (Covey, 1989)
- Some people will blame failures on uncontrollable forces like "the system."
- You can learn assertiveness skills to communicate more effectively and resolve conflicts without harming the integrity of others or yourself.

To speak assertively means to leave generalities behind. Address the details of the situation specifically, avoiding emotion-laden statements. Keeping to the facts of the matter will allow objective description of the issues. You can be clear and factual without hurting others.

Reactions and opinions should begin with "I" statements. Bower and Bower (1976) described the DESC format for formulating assertive responses. Use "I" statements to convey your point of view in a factual manner. Rather than "You" statements, which can feel accusatory, "I" statements suggest that the speaker assumes full responsibility for his or her position.

- Describe the situation—"The patient says that he did not receive..."
- Express your feelings about the situation—"I feel that ..."
- Specify that change or action that you want—"I would like for you to..."
- Consequences, identify the desired results—"In that way..."

It takes practice to use "I" statements routinely. With time and experience you will find that you can more effectively communicate for your patient and yourself. Assertiveness is an attribute that engenders respect from others because you can honestly state what is important and why.

CASE STUDY RESOLUTION

Juggling the many aspects of the job of nurse manager can be demanding. Rose thinks through the options: Tom could make one phone call to the transportation services, opiate medications must be delivered by a registered nurse in this state, and Tom needs to feel heard about how frustrating he is caring for this patient, particularly on a busy day.

Rose (nurse manager): "What a day! I am sorry that Mr. R. didn't get his pain medicine yet. It has been so busy. He's yelling at you again?"

Tom (nursing assistant): "Oh, yes. Can't you hear him? I seem to get assigned to him on the worst days."

Rose: "It must be hard dealing with him sometimes. I have an idea. What if you make this phone call and I'll bring Mr. R. his medication."

Tom: "Oh, I'll gladly make the call."

Rose: "How about we assign Mr. R. to someone else tomorrow?"

Tom: "I could use the break. Thanks."

EXERCISE

Practicing Assertiveness

Assertiveness is a skill that can be learned. Issues of sexism, power, and authority can make communicating assertively challenging. Read the following case study and discuss different ways the nurse could express herself. Decide as a group if the suggested responses are passive, aggressive, or assertive.

> *The nurse is standing at the nursing station on a medical-surgical floor of an acute care hospital. As she is reviewing the patient's chart, the surgeon walks up to her and says, "Honey, I am in a rush and I need that patient's chart right now." He sticks out his hand for her to hand the chart over. The nurse feels flustered and angry because she is not finished charting.*

How can the nurse respond?

Chapter 15

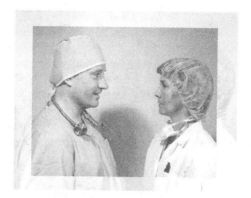

Conflict Resolution and Negotiation Skills

Case Study

When Mr. R. arrived on the medical-surgical floor, he was an active 67-year-old with peripheral arterial disease in need of an arterial bypass to restore circulation to his left leg. The pain in his left calf has been limiting his activities, especially his favorite pastime, gardening. Unfortunately, the graft became blocked 2 days after surgery. Now Mr. R. requires a below-the-knee amputation. Mr. R. is concerned about returning home after the surgery, as he is widowed and lives alone. Gail, his primary nurse, has finally found the surgeon and wants to discuss tentative discharge planning for Mr. R. She says, "Good morning, Dr. S., I want to talk with you about Mr. R.'s concerns about discharge." The surgeon replies, "Listen, I am really busy and you'll have to deal with this on your own. Can you get me his chart?"

INTRODUCTION

In human relationships, conflict is inevitable and often uncomfortable. In health care, the potential for conflict is heightened by the complexity of roles and issues. Life-altering decisions are made frequently that affect patients, their families, and the staff. But conflict is not necessarily bad, nor should it be avoided. While conflict often brings feelings of discomfort, frustration, and stress, it also brings opportunities for growth and change. Effective conflict resolution promotes positive outcomes, fosters connections between workers, and enhances job satisfaction.

CONFLICT RESOLUTION

The most common type of conflict in health care is interpersonal conflict: a conflict between individuals. The individuals might be coworkers or a patient and a nurse. In the case study, coworkers, the nurse and surgeon, are not communicating well about the patient, Mr. R. The nurse is using her role to advocate for the patient, and the surgeon does not see discharge planning as his role.

Conflict resolution between coworkers is an important part of maintaining and strengthening collaborative relationships. It is important to remember that most conflicts do not occur on an emergent basis. For example, the nurse might be asked to do something that feels unsafe or is spoken to in a condescending or hostile manner. A "cooling off" period allows for the emotional burden of the conflict to dissipate and for logical approaches to the conflict to be devised. Sometimes the most appropriate approach is "Let me get back to you later, after I have had some time to think about that." Interpersonal conflicts need to be dealt with in an effective manner to prevent lingering feelings that can interfere with future communication.

Frequently, dealing with authority figures is threatening to nurses. Real authority figures, like nursing managers, or perceived authority figures, like the surgeon in the case study, can intimidate younger or insecure nurses. The nurse needs to understand his or her personal feelings about authority before confronting authority figures with concerns. Be aware of the "inner voice," that part of the self that reacts emotionally. For example, if physicians intimidate the nurse, then it is acceptable to acknowledge this, but, at the same time, realize that it need not impede talking with the physician with a patient problem.

Dealing with interpersonal conflict in nurse-patient relationships can be challenging and often illuminating. For example, an elderly man is not taking his antihypertensive medication, and his blood pressure is high for the third visit. The nurse is frustrated because they have repeatedly discussed his need to take the medication, and on this visit his blood pressure is quite high. In the past, we called these patients "noncompliant," but what truly exists is a gap in communication. The nurse needs to evaluate the patient's reasons for not taking his medication, instead of labeling him as "noncompliant." On further questioning, the nurse learns that this patient is not taking his medication because of problems with impotence that he was afraid to discuss with a female nurse. When the source of his problem was identified, a new medication was ordered, with fewer effects on sexual functioning. Open communication allows the flexibility to explore problems and find solutions.

Identification of the actual problem is the beginning of creative problem solving and conflict resolution. Both parties need time to present their ideas, including possible solutions. When the involved parties feel "heard," then lingering feelings of resentment or manipulation are less likely to occur. Sometimes, writing down the issues on cards or going over the scenario with a trusted colleague will help with problem identification and diffusion of emotional content prior to discussion between the involved parties.

NEGOTIATION SKILLS

Using effective strategies to deal with conflict enhances positive outcomes and maintains the integrity of the participants. Negotiation skills are helpful in resolving conflicts and meeting the needs of the involved parties. Jones, Bushardt, and Caldenhead (1990) describe the use of **confrontation** to resolve conflicts. This is not confrontation in the aggressive sense, but the identification of concerns as a constructive means to reaching a solution. The four steps of confrontation described by Jones et al. are:
1. Identify concerns from involved parties.
2. Clarify assumptions.
3. Identify the real issue being confronted.
4. Work collaboratively to arrive at a mutually agreeable solution.

To identify the relevant concerns, the involved parties need time to organize their thoughts into a logical format. People have different communication styles. Some can handle interactions directly and decide on the spot how to resolve an issue. Others require time to process the information before the dialogue can continue.

Both parties bring assumptions to the conflict. In the case study at the beginning of the chapter, the nurse assumes that the surgeon is interested in participating in the discharge planning. The surgeon assumes that this part of patient care is within the nurse's province. Clarifying assumptions helps to establish not only differences, but also define common ground from which to begin negotiation. Assumptions can be fueled by emotion. In the case study, the nurse might feel that the surgeon is being condescending to her and uncaring toward the patient. Identifying and letting go of assumptions allows the actual problem to come into focus.

Self-confidence goes a long way toward promoting patient issues. Knowing the nurse's role, both in the institution and within the profession, helps you define your ability and power to make change. When unsure about the scope of nursing practice, you should refer to written guidelines (like a policy and procedures manual) or discuss the situation with a supervisor. Understanding the roles and expectations of the involved parties supports the nurse's position and stimulates self-confidence. It takes courage to confront those in authority. Do not let intimidation change what you want from the negotiation. A combination of professional guidelines and personal integrity allows you to present the facts in a knowledgeable and confident manner.

Problem solving requires negotiation between the involved parties. Negotiation strategies are used in business and health care to arrive at mutually agreeable solutions. Fisher, Ury, and Patton (1991) described four points to consider before entering negotiation.

1. Separate the people from the problem to depersonalize the negotiation what you are for and against.

2. Focus on interests—what you want to gain, not positions.

3. Invent options for mutual gain—a "win-win" solution.

4. Insist on objective—not emotional—criteria.

Negotiation is actually a combination of empathetic communication and creative cooperation. Covey (1989) described the process of trying to "understand first and then be understood" as empathetic communication. Using this process during negotiation allows the involved parties to be heard and arrive at mutually agreeable solutions. Covey also proposes that negotiation "begin with the end in mind." For example, if your ultimate goal is to have adequate home care in place prior to a patient's discharge, then that should be the focus of the discussion. Rarely does someone want to have "an end" that involves harsh words about another's personality. Negotiation is a process in which different viewpoints come together to make a single, mutually agreeable outcome.

Negotiation Strategies

- Set the stage. Meet at a set time in a private location, express a sincere desire to understand the issues, and show respect for the opinions of others.

- Establish points of agreement. Identify the common purpose and shared values and goals.

- Define the problem. Listen carefully, gather data, allow all parties to discuss concerns, and allow full disclosure of the issues.

- Be respectful of the participants. Avoid blaming, coercion, or intimidation.

- Analyze the problem. Paraphrase and using clarifying statements. ("Are you saying that...?" "If this happened instead, what would...?")
- Propose solutions. Be flexible; start from shared perspectives. ("We all want to see Mr. R. discharged home when he is able to care for himself.")

CONSTRUCTIVE CRITICISM OR FEEDBACK

Because giving and receiving constructive criticism is often difficult, it is frequently avoided. The word **feedback** is used to take away some of the negative connotation. Feedback provides the opportunity for exchange and promotes growth. Some strategies for giving and receiving feedback can make the communication a more positive experience. Given a non-threatening environment, participants can communicate more openly. A positive environment also maintains the dignity of the involved parties.

Giving Constructive Criticism

- Allow time for a "cooling-off" period if necessary.
- Set up a private time, free from patient responsibilities and other staff, to discuss the issue.
- Establish common values (e.g., safe patient care or timely medication administration).
- Express empathy for what the person is experiencing (e.g., "I know how short-staffed the floor is, and how difficult it is to complete your medications.").
- Describe the issue in factual terms ("Mr. R.'s pain medicine was an hour late, and he was uncomfortable.").
- State the expected behavior ("Medications need to be administered in a timely manner. Ask for help if you are having difficulty completing assignments.").
- Explain the consequences if the behavior continues ("Part of the expectation of your job is that medications be delivered to patients in a timely manner. If this happens again we will have to address it as part of your job evaluation.").

Receiving Constructive Criticism

- Allow the person (supervisor, peer, other health care provider) to voice his or her concerns.
- Do not let emotions cause overreactions.
- Discuss and paraphrase the issue so that both parties understand it.
- Respond to concerns with a serious intent to improve the situation.
- Develop a solution together to resolve the issue.

CASE STUDY RESOLUTION

Each person in this case had his or her own perspective. The primary nurse, Gail, is surprised by the surgeon's comments, as she assumed that the surgeon would want to talk about Mr. R.'s discharge. The surgeon is feeling rushed, because he has to get to the operating room for a case. He actually has a great deal of respect for Gail's abilities, but he is pressured by time and circumstance. Gail takes a deep breath, organizes her thoughts, and says: "I can see that you are busy right now. I have one more thing to document and then I can give you the chart. When would be a better time to talk about Mr. R.'s discharge planning?"

EXERCISE

Practicing Negotiation Skills

Learning to negotiate effectively improves communication. As a group, use assertiveness skills and the steps for negotiation to find a common solution for the problem presented in the following case study.

> Mrs. P. has been working the night shift at the nursing home for 8 months. She has three children at home and the arrangements for child care are becoming increasingly stressful. When she was hired, the supervisor told her that she would be switched to evenings within 6 months of starting work. Mrs. P. decides to approach the supervisor about the shift change. When she sees the supervisor coming out of a patient's room with the nurse manager, she says, "Excuse me, but I need to talk with you about changing my shift." Before she can say anymore, the supervisor says, "I really can't talk now. Can't you see that we have a crisis here?"

How will Mrs. P. pursue this?

Chapter *16*

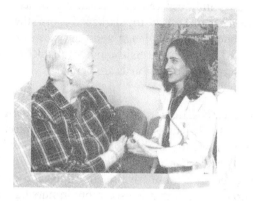

A CONCLUSION AND A BEGINNING

CASE STUDY

Theresa is a 72-year-old woman with non-small cell lung cancer whom we have been treating with intravenous chemotherapy for a year. She arrives with her husband of 51 years. The ongoing chemotherapy requires weekly venous access, often with multiple attempts. A port had to be removed because of thrombus formation. The available veins are small and very fragile. After two unsuccessful attempts at starting an intravenous line, Theresa, in her good-natured way, says, "We had better call in the professionals." The "professionals" to whom she refers are the intravenous nurses at the hospital. Because the I.V. team is short-staffed, it could be hours before Theresa would begin her long day of chemotherapy. Knowing that Theresa has a good sense of humor and trusts the nursing staff, the nurses decide to try one more time, but this time with special effects. "Theresa," I say, "If you will let us try one more time, we have one more trick up our sleeves. If this doesn't work, we will call in the professionals." The lights are turned off, and the nurses walk slowly across the room with the "vein-finder," the two-pronged lighted device often used to find deep veins in pediatric patients. As they approach Theresa with two dots of light in the darkened room, they make the sound of a drum roll. Theresa starts to laugh and concedes to one more try. This time, success! The I.V. line is in. As the nurses thank her for her patience, Theresa says, "I think the professionals are here."

The power of creative and effective nursing care is strengthened by good communication skills. Patients share their stories, symptoms, and concerns by talking with us. Both the spoken words and the body language convey information about the patient's experience. Your words can do so much: put a patient at ease, set up a productive relationship, and carry out interventions. There is no other skill that is used more in nursing than communication. Treating patients with honesty and respect, understanding their personalities, and putting their needs first can result in wonderful experiences that enrich the care of our patients and our lives as nurses.

When I was teaching nursing students in the clinical setting, it became apparent that many students were unsure about how to talk with patients. Often they focused on their skills sheet and tried to perfect their technical skills, like performing an intramuscular injection or a wet-to-dry dressing change. However, before any technical intervention can take place, communication begins between the nurse and patient. Meeting a new postoperative patient at the start of a shift, assessing a woman in labor, educating a patient about diabetes, setting treatment goals with a patient with breast cancer—all of these encounters begin with communication. And good communication skills are not only important for relaying information, they are essential for establishing trust and rapport, showing respect for the needs and feelings of others, and reaping the rewards of connecting with other people who just happen to be the patients in our care.

Each nurse enters the profession for different reasons, but I believe that the most frequent reason is because we enjoy caring for and working with other people. Now, when encounters with patients are limited by time constraints and workloads, it is even more important to condense the important aspects of good communication. This book is not meant to simplify a skill that is never truly perfected. It explores some basic aspects of communication that can be taught in nursing school. These beginning skills allow you as students to develop confidence in your abilities to communicate and then to evolve your own communication style over the following years of nursing practice. Good communication also enhances the nurse-patient relationship, making a better health care experience for the patient and a more rewarding career for the nurse.

Nurses have a unique position within the health care system. We communicate with patients for extended periods of time, allowing for more disclosure by the patient and more opportunities for understanding their needs. Nurses also have contact with other health care professionals: doctors, physical and occupational therapists, dieticians, and social workers, to name a few. We tend to be the "center" of communication between different departments and specialties. You can use assertiveness and negotiation skills to advocate for your patients. In this way, communication in nursing is unique, making it crucial in achieving good outcomes for our patients.

No one ever masters communication skills. We constantly learn from every patient encounter. Patients share so much of themselves with us. Sometimes we see the world from a new perspective in a way that changes us forever. Other times we laugh together about the absurdities of life. But mostly, we are allowed to be part of the patient's experience and permitted to make a difference in their health and well-being. How you use your communication skills will evolve with time and experience. Let your own personality shape how you talk with patients. You will have opportunities in nursing that few other jobs have—the ability to touch and improve the lives of others. What a wonderful and unique job—nursing!

BIBLIOGRAPHY

American Hospital Association. (1992). *A patient's bill of rights*. Chicago: Author.

American Nurses Association. (1973). *Standards of nursing practice*. Kansas City, MO: Author.

American Nurses Association. (1980). *Nursing: A social policy statement*. Kansas City, MO: Author.

American Nurses Association. (1991). *Standards of clinical nursing practice*. Kansas City, MO: Author.

American Nurses Association. (1976, 1985). *The code for nurses with interpretive statements*. Kansas City, MO: Author.

American Nurses Association. (2002). *Code of ethics for nurses*. Kansas City, MO: Author.

Andrews, M. M., & Boyle, J. S. (1997). Competence in transcultural nursing. *Am J Nurs, 97*(8), 16AAA-16DDD.

Andrews, M., & Boyle, J. (Eds.). (1999). *Transcultural concepts in nursing care* (3rd ed.). New York: Lippincott.

Arnold, E., & Boggs, K. U. (1999). *Interpersonal relationships: Professional communication skills for nurses*. Philadelphia: W. B. Saunders Co.

Baldwin, D. (January 31, 2003). Disparities in health and health care: Focusing care to eliminate unequal burdens. *Online Journal of Issues in Nursing, 8*(1), Manuscript 2. Retrieved November 10, 2003 from http://nursing-world.org/ojin/topic20/tpc20_1.htm

Bonder, B., Martin, L., & Miracle, A. (2002). *Culture in clinical care*. Thorofare, NJ: SLACK Incorporated.

Boucher, M. A. (1998). Delegation alert. *Am J Nurs, 98*(2), 26-33.

Bowen, M. (1985). *Family therapy in clinical practice*. Northvale, NJ: Jason Aronson.

Bower, S. A., & Bower, G. H. (1976). *Asserting yourself*. Reading, MA: Addison-Wesley.

Bowlby, J. (1980). *Attachment and loss: Loss, sadness and depression*. (Vol. 3). New York: Basic Books.

Campinha-Bacote, J. (January 31, 2003). Many faces: Addressing diversity in health care. *Online Journal of Issues in Nursing, 8*(1), Manuscript 2. Retrieved October 24, 2003 from http://nursingworld.org/ojin/topic20/tpc202.htm

Chavez, L. R., et. al. (1995). Understanding knowledge and attitudes about breast cancer: A cultural analysis. *Archives of Family Medicine, 4*, 145-152.

Collins, M. (1977). *Communication in health care*. St. Louis: The C. V. Mosby Co.

Cook, C. (January 31, 2003). The many faces of diversity: Overview and summary. *Online Journal of Issues in Nursing, 8*(1). Retrieved October 24, 2003 from http://nursingworld.org/ ojin/topic20/tpc20ntr.htm

Coulehan, J. L., & Block, M. R. (2001). *The medical interview*. Philadelphia: F. A. Davis Co.

Covey, S. R. (1989). *The 7 habits of highly effective people*. New York: Fireside.

Davis, C. M. (1998). *Patient practitioner interaction: An experiential manual for developing the art of health care* (3rd ed.). Thorofare, NJ: SLACK Incorporated.

Deering G.G., & Cody, D.J. (2002). Communicating with children and adolescents. *Am J Nurs, 2*(3), 31-41.

DeSantis, L. (1994). Making anthropology clinically relevant to nursing care. *J Adv Nurs, 20*, 707-715.

Edelman, C., & Mandle, C. L. (1994). *Health promotion throughout the life span* (3rd ed.). St. Louis, MO: Mosby-Year Book, Inc.

Erikson, E. (1963). *Childhood and society*. New York: Norton.

Erikson, E. (1981). *Life cycle completed*. New York: Norton.

Fawcett, J. (1975). The family as a living open system: An emerging conceptual framework for nursing. *Int Nurs Rev, 22*, 113.

Fink, S. (1986). *Crisis management: Planning for the inevitable*. Watertown, MA: American Medical Associates.

Fisher, R., Ury, W., & Patton, B. (1991). *Getting to yes: Negotiating agreement without giving in* (2nd ed.). Boston: Houghton-Mifflin.

Freud, S. (1937). *The basic writings of Sigmund Freud*. (A. A. Brill, trans./ed.). New York: Common Library.

Giger, J., & Davidhizar, R. (Ed.). (1999). *Transcultural nursing: Assessment and intervention* (3rd ed.). New York: Mosby.

Gomez, E. G., & Gullatte, M. (2002). *Advocacy in health care: Teaching patients, caregivers and professionals*. Pittsburgh, PA: Oncology Nursing Society.

Hasse, J., Britt, T., Coward, D., et. al. (1992). Simultaneous concept analysis of spiritual perspective, hope, acceptance and self-transcendence. *Image, 24*(2), 140-147.

Health Care Communication Group. (2001). *Writing, speaking & communication for health care professionals*. New Haven, CT: Yale University Press.

Hein, E. C. (1980). *Communication in nursing practice*. Boston: Little, Brown and Co.

Highfield, M. E., & Carson, C. (1983). Spiritual needs of patients: Are they recognized? *Cancer Nurs, 6*, 187-192.

Ignatavius, D. (1995). *Medical-surgical nursing: A nursing process approach*. Philadelphia: W. B. Saunders Co.

Itano, J. K., & Taoko, K. N. (1998). *Core curriculum for oncology nursing*. Philadelphia: W. B. Saunders Co.

Jones, M. A., Bushardt, S. C., & Caldenhead, G. (1990). A paradigm for effective resolution of interpersonal conflict. *Nursing Management, 21*, 64B.

Kazanowski, M. K., & Lacetti, M. S. (2002). *Pain.* Thorofare, NJ: SLACK Incorporated.

Keubler, K. K., Berry, P. H., & Heidrich, D. E. (2002). *End of life care: Clinical practice guidelines.* New York: W. B. Saunders Co.

King, I. M. (1971). *Toward a theory of nursing: General concepts of human behavior.* New York: Wiley.

King, I. M. (1981). *Theory for nursing: Systems concepts, process.* New York: Wiley.

Kubler-Ross, E. (1969). *On death and dying.* New York: MacMillan.

Kundahl, K. K. (2003). Cultural diversity: An evolving challenge to physician-patient relationship. *JAMA, 289*(1), 94.

Leninger, M. (1978). *Transcultural nursing: Concepts, theories and practices.* New York: Wiley.

Lipkin, G. S., & Cohen, R. G. (1992). *Effective approaches to patients' behavior.* New York: Springer Publishing.

Long, L., & Prophit, S. P. (1981). *Understanding/responding: A communication manual for nurses.* Monterey, CA: Wadsworth Health Sciences Division.

Luckmann, J. (2000). *Transcultural communication in health care.* Canada: Delmar Thomson Learning.

Maxfield, C. L., Pohl, J. M., & Colling, K. (2003). Advance directives: A guide for patient discussions. *Nurse Practitioner, 28*(5), 38-47.

McCaffery, M. (1968). *Nursing Practice Theories Related to Cognition, Bodily Pain, and Man-Environment Interactions.* Los Angeles: UCLA Student Store.

McCaffrey, M., & Passero, C. (1999). *Pain: Clinical manual* (2nd ed.). St. Louis, MO: Mosby.

Merriam-Webster's Collegiate Dictionary (10th ed.). (1996). Springfield, MA: Merriam-Webster, Inc.

Parad, H. (1990). *Crisis intervention: The practitioner's sourcebook for brief therapy.* Milwaukee, WI: Family International.

Peplau, H. E. (1952). *Interpersonal relations in nursing.* New York: Putnam.

Peplau, H. E. (1991). *Interpersonal relations in nursing.* New York: Springer.

Peplau, H. E. (1992). Interpersonal relations: A theoretical framework for application in nursing practice. *Nurs Sci Q, 5*(1), 13-18.

Peplau, H. E. (1997). Peplau's theory of interpersonal relations. *Nursing Science Quarterly, 10*(4), 162-167.

Piaget, J., & Inhelder, B. (1969). *The psychology of the child.* New York: Basic Books.

Piaget, J. (1972). *The child's conception of the world.* Savage, MD: Littlefield-Adams.

Pulcjaski, C., & Romer, A. L. (2000). Taking a spiritual history allows clinicians to understand patients more fully. *J Palliat Med, 3*(1), 129-137.

Richmond, V., McCroskey, J., & Payne, S. (1987). *Nonverbal behavior in interpersonal relations*. Englewood Cliffs, NJ: Prentice-Hall.

Robinson, V. M. (1991). *Humor and the health professions*. Thorofare, NJ: SLACK Incorporated.

Rogers, C. (1951). *Client-centered therapy*. Boston: Houghton-Mifflin.

Rogers, C. (1961). *On becoming a person*. Boston: Houghton-Mifflin.

Rosenstock, I. M. (1974). Historical origins of the Health Belief Model. *Health Education Monographs, 2*(4), 354-386.

Rungapadiachy, D. M. (1999). *Interpersonal communication and psychology for health care professionals: Theory and practice*. Boston: Butterworth/ Heinemann.

Servonsky, J., & Opas, S. R. (1987). *Nursing management of children*. Boston: Jones & Bartlett.

Stuart, G. W., & Sundeen, S. J. (1991). *Principles and practice of psychiatric nursing* (4th ed.). St. Louis, MO: Mosby.

Sullivan, H. (1953). *The interpersonal theory of psychiatry*. New York: Norton.

Sundeen, S. J., et. al. (1994). *Nurse-client interaction: Implementing the nursing process* (5th ed.). St. Louis, MO: C. V. Mosby.

Travelbee, J. (1971). *Interpersonal aspects of nursing*. Philadelphia: F. A. Davis Co.

Turncock, C. (1991). Communicating with patients in the ICU. *Nursing Standards, 9*(5), 38-40.

U. S. Bureau of Census. (1990). *Social and economic characteristics*. Washington, DC: U. S. Government Printing Office.

U. S. Bureau of Census. (2000). *Statistical abstract of the United States*. Washington, DC: U. S. Government Printing Office.

U. S. Bureau of Census. Table PCT1: Total population. In: American Factfinder: 2000.

U. S. Center for Immigration Studies. *Census Bureau population survey for March 1998*. Los Angeles.

U. S. Department of Health and Human Services—Office of Civil Rights. (1996). *Health Insurance Portability and Privacy Act of 1996 (HIPPA)*. Retrieved October 24, 2003 from http://www.hhs.gov/ ocr/hipaa

Watson, J. (1995). Postmodernism and knowledge development in nursing. *Nurs Sci Q.* 8(2): 60, 1995.

Watzlawick, P., Beavin, J., & Jackson, D. D. (1967). *Pragmatics of human communication*. New York: Norton.

Worden, J. W. (1991). *Grief counseling and grief therapy: A handbook for the mental health practitioner* (2nd ed.). New York: Springer Publishing Co.

INDEX